**Brain Tumor
Chemotherapy**

Brain Tumor Chemotherapy

By

DEREK FEWER, M.D., CM., FRCS(C)

Lecturer, Department of Surgery
University of Manitoba Medical School
Associate Neurosurgeon, St. Boniface General Hospital
Winnipeg, Manitoba, Canada

CHARLES B. WILSON, M.D.

Professor and Chairman, Department of Neurological Surgery
Director, Brain Tumor Research Center, H.C. Naffziger Laboratories
Research Associate, Cancer Research Institute
University of California School of Medicine, San Francisco

VICTOR A. LEVIN, M.D.

Assistant Professor of Neurology, Neurosurgery, and
  Pharmaceutical Chemistry (School of Pharmacy)
Assistant Director, Brain Tumor Research Center
H.C. Naffziger Laboratories

With Contributions by

Marvin Barker, M.S.
Takao Hoshino, M.D.
K. Jean Enot, R.N.

RC280
B7
F48
1976

With a Foreword by

Edwin B. Boldrey, M.D.

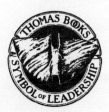

CHARLES C THOMAS • PUBLISHER
Springfield • Illinois • U.S.A.

Published and Distributed Throughout the World by
CHARLES C THOMAS ● PUBLISHER
Bannerstone House
301-327 East Lawrence Avenue, Springfield, Illinois, U.S.A.

© *1976, by* CHARLES C THOMAS ● PUBLISHER

ISBN 0-398-03549-0

Library of Congress Catalog Card Number: 75-46546

With THOMAS BOOKS *careful attention is given to all details of
manufacturing and design. It is the Publisher's desire to present books that are
satisfactory as to their physical qualities and artistic possibilities and
appropriate for their particular use.* THOMAS BOOKS *will be true to those
laws of quality that assure a good name and good will.*

Printed in the United States of America
R-1

Library of Congress Cataloging in Publication Data

Fewer, Derek
  Brain tumor chemotherapy.

  Bibliography: p.
  Includes index.
  1. Brain--Cancer--Chemotherapy. I. Wilson,
Charles B., 1929- joint author. II. Levin,
Victor A., joint author. III. Title. [DNLM:
1. Brain neoplasms--Drug therapy. WL358 F432b]
RC280.B7F48   616.9′94′81   75-46546
ISBN 0-398-03549-0

CONTRIBUTORS

MARVIN BARKER, M.S.

Associate Director, Brain Tumor Research Center
University of California
School of Medicine, San Francisco, California

K. JEAN ENOT, R.N.

Coordinator, Chemotherapy Service
Brain Tumor Research Center
University of California
School of Medicine, San Francisco, California

DEREK FEWER, M.D., CM., FRCS(C)

Lecturer, Department of Surgery
University of Manitoba Medical School
Associate Neurosurgeon, St. Boniface General Hospital
Winnipeg, Manitoba, Canada

TAKAO HOSHINO, M.D., D.M.Sc.

Assistant Professor of Neurosurgery
Brain Tumor Research Center
University of California
School of Medicine, San Francisco, California

VICTOR A. LEVIN, M.D.

Assistant Professor of Neurology, Neurosurgery, and
Pharmaceutical Chemistry
Assistant Director, Brain Tumor Research Center
University of California Schools of Medicine and Pharmacy
San Francisco, California

CHARLES B. WILSON, M.D.

Professor and Chairman
Department of Neurosurgery, University of California
Director, Brain Tumor Research Center
School of Medicine, San Francisco, California

DEDICATION

To our patients, the many colleagues who referred them, and the nursing personnel whose patience and understanding have been essential to this undertaking, we dedicate this book with affection and gratitude.

FOREWORD

SIGNIFICANT INTEREST AND success in the treatment of primary tumors of the brain is a phenomenon of the Twentieth Century — though based initially on studies of neoplasia and of form and function of the nervous system developed and pursued in the latter part of the Nineteenth. Three phases can be recognized. For the first three decades surgical methods grew from feeble sprouts to maturity and provided the sole, albeit usually dim, hope for those afflicted. During the next third of the century radiation therapy blossomed to join surgery usually in an adjunctive way, in selected circumstances, as the therapeutic method of choice. Chemotherapy is now beginning to take its place as a third line in man's defense against this terrifying adversary. At the present, it is usually adjunctive to surgical intervention, and for that matter, irradiation. There are notable examples, though, where chemotherapy may be chosen as the primary treatment, as in the case of unbiopsied brain tumors.

The surgical treatment of brain tumors progressed concomitantly with surgery in general; so in a similar fashion did radiation therapy. With chemotherapy, while there have been close ties with the evolution of the neurosciences, progress in the two fields has not been closely interrelated.

General oncologists have found the tumors of the brain, inaccessible as they are to ready inspection and to easy evaluation of results, to be less attractive subjects than the numerous other forms of cancer which could be explored in a more gratifying fashion. This reluctance has decreased with the development of analytical techniques such as isotope scanning, but aversion nevertheless persists.

Neurologists and neurological surgeons, although recognizing the potential of controlled cytocidal agents, have been slow as a group in objective willingness to devote the time, thought, and

ix

energy required for the effective exploitation of these agents. The difficulty has not been entirely one of indifference. Few areas in the world have adequate numbers of suitable patients, skilled diagnostic personnel, and facilities for both pre- and postoperative study. Basic research scientists are needed to provide adequately tested drugs of enough potential value to warrant use even in the grim circumstances under investigation. The public must be informed and enlightened; there must be lay as well as general professional personnel, including specialized nursing staff and skilled personnel to maintain continued communication with the profession as well as with the patients. Also, there must be financial support for the whole endeavor. Happily, such a constellation has been assembled, and a preliminary report of accomplishment is herewith presented.

Even with such an assembly, periodic evaluation of ongoing success or failure has been a major difficulty for students of intracranial neoplasia. It has been necessary to develop methods whereby at least some aspects of tumor behavior can be followed sequentially. Angiography, scintiphoto isotope scanning, and perhaps computerized axial tomography now make this a reasonable possibility.

The remaining "Achilles' heel" of chemotherapy is the hematopoietic system. This challenge is among the more major ones remaining.

Chemotherapy of brain tumors represents another step toward an ultimate goal of cure. A few intracranial neoplasms can be eliminated by anatomical removal (surgery); a few more by complete differential destruction through physiological means (irradiation); chemotherapy involves cytotoxic agents to attack still others. The ultimate cure of a malady rests with the creation of an intrinsic self-preserving mechanism by the whole organism. This defense must be able to overwhelm remaining elements of an aggressive intruder, even one *sui generis*. All else may be regarded as ancillary, succeeding only when the complex natural mechanism of immunity can destroy all dangerous elements that remain, regardless of location. This happy circumstance now seems to be a real possibility, in view of the rapid advances in several related areas. The approaches described by the contributors to this unique volume represent some of the most promising aspects of this multidimensional effort to bring malignant brain tumors under complete therapeutic control.

EDWIN B. BOLDREY, M.D.

PREFACE

During the last decade, interest in the chemotherapy of solid tumors has reached an all-time high. Chemotherapeutic success in acute childhood leukemia, choriocarcinoma, and Burkitt's lymphoma has evoked unprecedented optimism in the search for new and more effective oncolytic agents. No less promising are studies exploring more effective schedules for administering agents known to possess activity. For the first time, knowledge of tumor cell population kinetics and crucial experiments in animal models have indicated what was suspected but unproved. In the past, an agent was pushed to toxicity with the hope that it would achieve selective toxicity for the tumor cell population while sparing normal tissues. The critical role of drug schedules can be questioned no longer, and many laboratory and clinical studies indicate clearly that selective toxicity is achieved, not by unique vulnerability of the cancer cell, but by selective toxicity based upon differences in the kinetic parameters of normal and neoplastic cells. With little doubt this represents one of the great achievements of the past decade and clearly points to the wave of the future.

After the introduction of radionuclide imaging techniques, most chemotherapists assumed that intracerebral tumors possessed no barrier to many substances excluded by the normal blood-brain barrier, and as a consequence little effort was extended in the direction of exploiting agents capable of penetrating the intact blood-brain barrier. In the chapter on pharmacology the rationale for favoring the use of nitrosoureas and other drugs with similar permeability characteristics is explained. For each drug there exists an optimal method of administration, i.e., route of delivery, dose, and schedule. First priority may not be the discovery of new agents but rather the optimal use of drugs currently available.

xiii

In the past two years we have gained additional experience in conducting Phase II drug trials, and this represents our major effort. The Brain Tumor Study Group, of which we are a member, has now completed one Phase III study and a second study is in the final stages of analysis. This represents an enormous advance but is less impressive when one compares it to the many completed protocols involving nonneural solid tumors. The several solid tumor cooperative groups have ignored primary brain tumors, and the few cooperative studies involving metastatic tumors have yielded limited information. We hope that brain tumor chemotherapeutic trials can be instituted to encompass a larger population of patients, and the best mechanism for such an effort would seem to be a cooperative arrangement between the Brain Tumor Study Group and other cooperative groups.

In this monograph we have summarized the information available at the present time. We hope that this volume will become obsolete within a short time, and this we predict. Much of our material has been taken from the work of others. In particular, we express a debt of gratitude and a deep sense of appreciation to Dr. David Rall, whose influence played such a major role in the evolution of the Brain Tumor Study Group, and in the junior author's education in the pharmacokinetics of cancer chemotherapy.

We undertook this task recognizing our own limitations, yet believing that a monograph at this stage of our knowledge would serve to summarize accomplishments thus far and stimulate further work.

CHARLES B. WILSON, M.D.
June, 1976

ACKNOWLEDGMENTS

DAVID RALL, STEVEN CARTER, and Michael Walker of the NCI for encouragement and advice.

Glenn Sheline and Theodore Phillips for close cooperation in problems related to chemotherapy.

Malcolm Powell for establishing criteria for evaluation by radionuclide imaging.

T. Hans Newton and a succession of Neuroradiology Fellows for assistance in interpreting diagnostic studies.

Surl Nielsen for reviewing all of the pathologic material.

Harvey Patt and James Cleaver for advice regarding kinetic studies.

Robert Elashoff for statistical consultation.

Margaret Sucec and Gretchen Limper, the editors, for their patience with the authors.

Deborah Morgan who typed countless drafts and the final copy.

The authors wish to acknowledge the sources of various grants which supported this project.

Brain Tumor Research Center
National Institutes of Health
Ca. 13525

Pharmacokinetics of Brain Tumor Chemotherapy
National Institutes of Health
Ca. 15435

A gift from Phi Beta Psi Sorority

A gift from Joe Gheen Medical Foundation

A gift from the Association for Brain Tumor Research

D.F.
C.B.W.
V.A.L.

CONTENTS

Brain Tumor
Chemotherapy

CHAPTER **ONE**

CHEMOTHERAPY — HISTORY AND GENERAL CONSIDERATIONS

DEREK FEWER

THIS BOOK IS intended for neurologists and neurosurgeons who have had little or no experience with clinical chemotherapy; it is, therefore, appropriate to begin by answering some obvious and fundamental questions about this form of treatment. This chapter will briefly review the history of cancer chemotherapy, trace the usual course of development and testing of a chemotherapeutic agent today, and discuss briefly two basic research discoveries which have been important in establishing appropriate schedules for the clinical use of chemotherapeutic agents.

HISTORY OF CANCER CHEMOTHERAPY[1]

The first compounds tested for antitumor activity were obtained from a variety of sources, mostly unconnected with cancer, and included antibiotics derived from bacterial fermentation, natural products from plants, and synthesized chemicals. When some of these compounds showed antitumor activity in animals, screening programs were established in several centers to determine the basis for this activity and to obtain more active agents. These original screening tests were an offshoot of research carried out as part of the war effort between 1940 and 1945, and were made possible by the prewar development of several animal tumors in inbred rats in which antitumor agents could be tested.

In the decade following the Second World War, about 20,000 compounds were submitted for testing. The majority of this work was conducted at the Sloan-Kettering Institute. At this stage, animal screenings far surpassed clinical applications, as there were very few centers geared for clinical trials. Along with the increased numbers of compounds available for testing, new animal tumor

3

models were developed, including the carcinogen-induced L1210, which has become one of the most useful, predictable models available today.

The Cancer Chemotherapy National Service Center (CCNSC) was created in 1955 by the National Cancer Institute to coordinate drug development and testing, and more important, to sponsor, activate, and coordinate cooperative clinical screening studies on a national level. The CCNSC provided leadership in the fields of organic chemistry, drug screening, pharmacology, biochemistry, documentation, and biometry.

Among the first actions of CCNSC was the expansion of animal-breeding and animal-testing facilities to accommodate the increasing numbers of products submitted for screening. It was estimated that only one drug out of every thousand tested would reach clinical trial. CCNSC also designed and implemented methods for data processing, storage, and retrieval, which have been modified and improved over the years. Within three years of its formation, the chemotherapy program required a $35 million budget to sustain its extensive activities.

Zubrod, et al. describes the CCNSC chemotherapy program by 1959 as "an industrial drug development program funded through contracts, coupled with a loosely coordinated clinical trial apparatus, self-generated in many instances, and funded entirely through research grants."[1] With the operation now so large, research efforts within each of the major CCNSC subdivisions were coordinated by separate advisory panels, based on the feedback of data from the entire project. As drug-screening experience was gained in animal systems, rigid statistical parameters for conducting the studies and interpreting their results were established and accepted. New screening methods, such as cell culture cytotoxicity tests, were developed, evaluated, and found to correlate acceptably with *in vivo* results; criteria for their use were established and implemented. Until 1960, only three animal tumor systems were used for screening; this was then expanded to a group of twenty tumors. Each agent screened was tested in at least three of the available systems.

Many clinical studies had been completed by the early 1960's. Although the overall results were considered disappointing, findings for some drugs against a number of tumors were encouraging. For this reason, the efforts of the chemotherapy program were reoriented with greater emphasis on the biology and treatment of specific tumors in the hope that increased understanding of the basic principles of tumor growth would yield a more rational approach to practical chemotherapy.

Brain Tumor Study Group

By the mid-1960's only sporadic individual efforts had been made to use chemotherapeutic agents against tumors in the brain, and none of these had statistically proven or disproven the value of any given drug. Those interested in brain tumor chemotherapy realized that only through collaboration could they initiate clinical trials involving significant numbers of patients. Representatives from five university neurosurgical departments, the National Cancer Institute, and the National Institute of Neurological Diseases and Blindness met in 1966 to form the Brain Tumor Chemotherapy Study Group (BTCSG). The university departments provided the base for clinical research, supported by funds from the National Cancer Institute.

The original aim was to adopt common protocols and pool results in order to complete studies within a reasonable period of time. Three such studies have been designed up to now: Two involving mithramycin and carmustine (BCNU) have been completed, and the third, involving MeCCNU, (methyl-C-1-(2 chloroethyl)-3-cyclohexyl-1-nitrosourea), is now in progress.

DRUG DEVELOPMENT — THE "LINEAR ARRAY"

In current research, all chemotherapeutic agents are put through a standard series of steps to determine their potential for clinical application. Drugs submitted for screening are no longer proposed at random; the structure-activity relationships of most classes of agents in current clinical or experimental practice are recognized and efforts are made to synthesize analogs of these known structures. In addition, new classes of agents are sought which are considered potentially useful in the light of increasing understanding of the biochemical and kinetic mechanisms of cancer cell activity.

Initially, the chemical structure of the pure drug is identified, and its physical characteristics are determined (i.e., chemical stability, solubility, etc.). This determination is an important prerequisite for preparing a form of the agent suitable for *in vivo* administration.

The drug is then tested in one or more small animal screening systems. These systems consist of inbred strains of rats or mice bearing tumors, originally induced or arising spontaneously, transplantable to successive generations with a high percentage of tumor "takes". The tumor growth characteristics of these animal systems are well defined, with a relatively short life expectancy after tumor implantation (usually about thirty days). In most screening procedures, a positive antitumor effect is identified on the basis of an increased life span compared to that of an untreated control group. Several methods have been standardized for conducting these studies (i.e., in dose selection, schedules of administration, and evaluation of results); these methods have been reviewed in an excellent paper by Goldin.[2]

After initial studies have been completed, an agent is considered for further testing on three bases: (1) It shows significant antitumor activity; (2) it can be produced economically in substantial quantities; and (3) it demonstrates favorable structural characteristics, e.g., solubility. If a drug meets these criteria, it is then administered to tumor-free dogs and monkeys for qualitative and quantitative determination of its major organ toxicity and maximum tolerated dose. The organ function of dogs and monkeys is more closely analogous to that of humans than is the organ function of rodents. In a retrospective study in which dosage was calculated on a mg/m^2 of body surface basis, the qualitative and quantitative aspects of organ toxicity were almost identical in man and these larger animals.[3,4] Further testing in small animals then establishes schedules for maximum correlation between dose and drug activity. These experiments have yielded reproducible schedules for optimal dosage in human trials. If there are no projected difficulties with production, drug evaluation then proceeds to clinical trials.

Clinical studies are classically divided into Phases I, II, and III.[5,6] The criteria for selecting patients for each of these phases will be described in Chapter Five. In Phase I studies the objective is to establish a maximum tolerable dose for each of one or more different schedules of administration and to assess major organ toxicity and its degree of reversibility. The practical methodology for such a study has been reviewed by Holland.[7] A Phase I study is not intended to monitor antitumor effect, since the drug is evaluated in a random heterogeneous population of cancer patients. Nonetheless, such an effect is frequently observed; should the drug be considered for Phase II studies, these findings will be pertinent in determining which tumors are selected for study with the particular agent.

A Phase II study is designed to identify at least some antitumor activity in a homogeneous population of patients with a single tumor type and disease which has progressed to the extent that the tumor mass is measurable. This latter point is important, since the objective measurement of tumor growth or reduction is currently the most reliable index of a drug's usefulness. However, the location of many tumor types is such that even well-advanced growth cannot be easily defined in quantitative terms; malignant brain tumors fall into this latter group. In these cases, assessment of drug efficacy will be based on judgments of clinical response rather than on attempts at actual measurement of tumor size. This point will be elaborated further in Chapter Five.

A Phase III study is controlled and prospective. By the time a drug reaches Phase III testing, its toxicity has been determined, an optimal dose and schedule have been established, and a degree of antitumor activity against one or more tumor types has been demonstrated. Thus in a Phase III study chemotherapy is used, either alone or combined with surgery and/or radiotherapy in the initial definitive treatment of one specific form of malignancy. The criterion for response is usually considered to be an increase in the life span (ILS) of the treated patients compared to that of an untreated control group. In most instances, the percent ILS of a known, effective agent can be used as the lower limit of acceptability; that is, if the drug being tested does not produce a higher percent ILS, it will not be considered for further use. If a drug should offer other advantages over the known agent, e.g., a reduced or different form of toxicity or a different mechanism of action, a lower degree of effectiveness may be acceptable because the new agent may be valuable when used in combination with other drugs against a particular tumor. The same rationale can be applied to results in Phase II studies.

At present, the overall plan of the chemotherapy section of the National Cancer Institute for handling new drugs which reach the Phase II stage is to test each agent against six "signal" tumor types. These are: adenocarcinoma of the colon, adenocarcinoma of the breast, bronchogenic carcinoma, acute lymphatic leukemia, acute myelocytic leukemia and poorly differentiated malignant lymphoma. These types (a) are common and (b) cover the range of observed growth rates of human tumors. A drug which is effective in one or more of these signal systems is then considered for Phase III testing against the same tumor type or against a tumor with similar growth characteristics. A drug which shows defined, significant activity in a Phase III study can thereafter be regarded as an acceptable means of primary therapy for the tumor studied. By 1971 the chemotherapy program had made available through this complex testing system forty active drugs which represent twenty-four different chemical structures.[8]

Over the past decade, this schema or "linear array" has evolved continuously, and the length of time required for a drug to pass through it is much shorter now than ten years ago. To relate this to an agent used against brain tumors, for example, BCNU was developed at the Southern Research Institute in 1961 and entered Phase III testing in 1969. At the present time, clinical testing requires a minimum of about three years.

Some Aspects of Protocol Design

The significance of results from both Phase II and III testing depends primarily upon the quality of protocol design. Statistics assume a role of vital importance in protocol design if one is to arrive at valid conclusions, especially when comparing various treatment groups. In general, ten to twenty patients in each group of the study will suffice. The size of these groups can be more accurately determined according to methods described by Gehan.[9] Every effort must be made to eliminate or control major variables in the treated groups. If this is impossible then the study must be set up with as many groups as there are major variables, each containing a significant number of patients.

For example, patients who have malignant gliomas (astrocytoma grades three and four or glioblastoma multiforme) should not be included in the same treatment group as patients with more slowly growing gliomas (astrocytoma grades one and two), since the life expectancies for the two are so disparate. Similarly, patients who may have histologically identical tumors, but some of whom have received previous chemotherapy without response and some have not, are not comparable and thus should not be included in the same group. This latter point is becoming increasingly important in the chemotherapy of some cancers for which there already exists a drug with a proven beneficial effect (e.g., 5-fluorouracil Roche® (5-FU) for cancer of the colon). Many patients arriving at chemotherapy centers have already received one or more drugs. These patients are frequently prone to greater toxic side-effects (usually hematological) and therefore may not tolerate as much of the new agent as would untreated patients. More important, the fact that a previous chemotherapeutic attack on the tumor has occurred, with the patient either not responding at all or responding for a variable period and then failing to respond further, places a bias on a group of such patients. These already treated tumors may be much less responsive to any form of chemotherapy than tumors in untreated patients, since the prior treatment selectively killed all sensitive cells, leaving a drug-resistant clone of tumor cells as the dominant growth.

Previous radiation therapy places a similar therapeutic bias on a patient group. Other factors that may be important in treatment studies of certain tumors include age, sex, extent of previous surgery, length of time between initial treatment and recurrence, etc. Again, to emphasize the point, patient selection within the study is a critical factor, and patients must be stratified according to the major variables.

One practical point to note in the evaluation of patients who are receiving chemotherapy is that one should not be too hasty to label a patient as a failure. Responses have been seen in patients with malignant gliomas beginning as late as ten weeks after the time of initial treatment.

A theoretical argument against the concept of the Phase II study is that the ideal time for the most effective chemotherapeutic treatment has passed by the time a tumor has reached a symptomatic and measurable size, as has been shown by *in vivo* animal studies.[10] Thus, the best clinical screen for a drug is really the Phase III study, although this is also the definitive prospective test. The author agrees with the argument but is willing to accept the less-than-optimal circumstances in Phase II screening of agents for two main reasons. First, it is known now, in retrospect, that drug effectiveness can indeed be shown against brain tumors in a Phase II study,[11] and that the results obtained in such studies correlate well with findings from screenings in animals bearing brain tumors. There are probably exceptions to this rule because drugs that have proven effective in Phase II studies have all been cycle-specific agents (see discussion of Bruce's work below). Such drugs are theoretically active against a larger percentage of viable tumor cells than a phase-specific agent, such as Methotrexate.® Second, the limited availability of patients with brain tumors suitable for Phase III studies significantly prolongs the time required for adequate testing of a drug. For example, six university centers in the Brain Tumor Study Group combined their efforts for more than three years in order to gather enough patients for a well-designed Phase III study of BCNU against malignant gliomas. By comparison, a single referral institution can complete a Phase II study within one year.

All three of the studies carried out by the Brain Tumor Chemotherapy Study Group (mithramycin, BCNU, methyl-CCNU) have been designed as Phase III studies, since it was difficult for the group to agree on all of the criteria necessary for collaborative Phase II studies. Nevertheless, a number of the neurosurgical departments involved in BTCSG have designed and carried out their own individual Phase II studies.

The commonly used animal tumor screens involve intraperitoneal or subcutaneous sites of growth and consequently are poor models for predicting the value of a drug against brain tumors.

Mice bearing intracerebrally implanted L1210 leukemia represent an exception. The unique locus of brain tumors requires a similarly situated animal tumor that will mimic the growth and response to treatment of human brain tumors in a clinical situation.

BASIC PRINCIPLES OF CHEMOTHERAPY

In addition to research aimed at developing and evaluating individual drugs, research leading to the formulation of basic principles has been of enormous importance in the evolution of effective chemotherapy. These principles have grown out of concurrent observations in the study of normal and tumor cell kinetics, the pharmacologic disposition of chemotherapeutic agents *in vivo*, and empirical studies on both beneficial and toxic proper-ties of drugs used in animal screens. Some basic research in the common animal tumor models has influenced knowledge of tumor growth and the way chemotherapeutic treatment is applied, and has led to a new and useful classification of antitumor agents.

One basic but important observation is that anticancer agents affect all proliferating tissues. No drug used in clinical chemotherapy today has a specific effect on tumor cells alone; anticancer agents will injure the dividing components of the gastrointestinal epithelium, hair follicles, and most important, the bone marrow, since these tissues have the most rapid cell turnover in a normal vertebrate system. With few exceptions, e.g., bleomycin and vincristine, bone marrow toxicity, that is, destruction of the dividing bone marrow precursor cells with subsequent reduction of formed cells (leukocytes, platelets, and red cells) in the peripheral circulation, becomes the dose-limiting factor in chemotherapy. This observation was made quite early in clinical chemotherapy, and led to searches for nonhemotoxic drugs and attempts to modify the schedules of administration to gain therapeutic advantage. The latter approach has been more productive. In defining the basis for optimal drug schedules, understanding of the basic principles of tumor growth has increased considerably.

In 1956 Goldin, et al. demonstrated that different schedules of maximally tolerated doses of Methotrexate dramatically influenced the survival of mice bearing L1210 leukemia.[12] Subsequently, virtually every drug in use has been found to demonstrate schedule dependency. A representative sample of such data was reported by Skipper, et al.[13] Differences in the kinetic characteristics of normal and neoplastic cell populations provide the basis for schedule dependency.

The life and reproduction of any viable cell can be divided into four (possibly five) phases because of specific biochemical events taking place in each phase.[14] The definitions of these phases, established by various radioisotopic techniques, are found in the next chapter ("Cell Cycle Kinetics", Chapter Two). Normal and tumor cells, both *in vivo* and *in vitro*, have been investigated, and the duration of each phase, and thus of the whole cell cycle, has been determined. In similar experiments *in vitro*, chemotherapeutic agents have been added to normal and tumor cell cultures, and the phase or phases during which the agents have inhibited cell growth have been determined.

In 1964 Skipper, et al.[15] published a monumental paper on experimental chemotherapy of the rapidly proliferating L1210 leukemia in mice. Their observations confirmed and extended the observations of Goldin.[12] Both groups showed that intermittent, high dose therapy (given at the maximally tolerated dose and repeated when toxicity had subsided), was the optimal treatment schedule. Skipper showed that the percent of leukemia cell kill after a single dose was directly proportional to the size of the dose. He concluded: "Since most antileukemic agents are, to a considerable degree, cumulative in their toxicity to experimental animals, and since the proliferation of surviving leukemia cells rapidly replaces partial cell kill achieved by necessarily relatively low chronic doses, it appears that high dose intermittent schedules offer considerably greater potential for obtaining cures."[13]

The question now arose: Why did doses and schedules leading to a marked increase in life span not, in fact, kill the animals from marrow depression? The answer came from the work of Bruce and his colleagues, who used another rapidly proliferating animal model, the AKR lymphoma.[16] They developed a spleen colony bioassay[17] which allows a parallel assessment of the effects of the anticancer agent on both the normal marrow and the tumor cell population. In testing many oncolytic agents they identified three characteristic survival curves. These curves define three specific types of drug action. The shape of these response curves for both normal and malignant cells can be explained by postulating that a particular drug is active against : (1) cells in a specific phase of the cell cycle (phase-specific), (2) cells in all phases of the cell cycle (cycle-specific), or (3) cells both in and out of cycle (cycle-nonspecific). The authors of this book recognize this classification of antitumor agents as more meaningful (because it is functional) than those in current use, and will use it throughout this book.

The most important observation of Bruce and his colleagues was a quantitative difference in the slope of dose response curves for normal marrow stem cells and malignant cells following exposure to both phase-specific and cycle-specific agents. A logical explanation for this difference is that fewer marrow stem cells than lymphoma cells are proliferating at any one time (see Chapter Two). Consequently, fewer stem cells are susceptible to destruction by cycle-specific and phase-specific agents. Thus, for patients with otherwise normal marrow function, it is possible to obtain a therapeutic advantage — more with rapidly growing tumors, less with slowly growing tumors (e.g., solid tumors) — using intermittent, high dose treatment schedules.

In practical terms, Bruce's experiments indicate that a phase-specific agent should be maintained at effective dose levels for a period at least as long as one generation time to achieve maximum kill of proliferating cells as they cycle through the particular phase, while for the cycle-specific agents, single high dose but intermittent therapy is the ideal schedule. The choice of drug doses and schedules for Phase II or Phase III protocols at the present time is based on these principles. When various doses and schedules of arabinosyl cytosine were administered to patients with a variety of metastatic tumors, the dose response vs. toxicity results correlated well with those that Bruce found using the same agent against the AKR lymphoma.[18]

The above work has not been repeated in brain tumor systems, but until results to the contrary are shown in such systems, the author believes that the principles formulated as a result of this work can supply the guidelines for brain tumor chemotherapy. In addition, the recent heightened interest in brain tumor chemotherapy has led to the use of animal brain tumor models as research tools. Brain tumor models have filled many of the gaps in areas where the treatment of central nervous system tumors differs from the treatment of tumors in other locations. This will be discussed more fully in Chapter Four. First, however, the vital basic work being done in the areas of tumor cell growth kinetics and pharmacokinetics will be examined in more detail.

REFERENCES

1. Zubrod, C.G., Schepartz, S., Leiter, J., et al.: The chemotherapy program of the National Cancer Institute: history, analysis, and plans. *Cancer Chemother Rep, 50*:348, 1966.
2. Goldin, A.: Preclinical methodology for the selection of anticancer agents. In Busch, H. (Ed.): *Methods of Cancer Research*, New York, Acad Pr, 1968, vol. IV, chapt. VII, pp. 193-254.
3. Freireich, E., Gehan, E., Rall, D., et al.: Quantitative comparison of toxicity of anticancer agents in mouse, rat, and hamster, dog, monkey, and man. *Cancer Chemother Rep, 50*:219, 1966.
4. Schein, P., Davis, R., Carter, S., et al.: The toxicologic evaluation of anticancer drugs in dogs and monkeys as a basis for the prediction of quantitative toxicities in man. *Proc Am Assoc Cancer Res, 10*:76, 1969.
5. Brindley, C.: Methodology of preliminary chemotherapeutic trials in patients with malignant solid tumors. *Cancer Chemother Rep, 32*:27, 1963.
6. Carter, S.: From a paper presented at the Second Joint Working Conference, National Cancer Institute Chemotherapy Program, Annapolis, Maryland, November 3-5, 1971.
7. Holland, J.: Methods in cancer chemotherapy research in man. In Busch, H. (Ed.): *Methods in Cancer Research*, New York, Acad Pr, 1968, vol. IV, chapt. VIII, pp. 255-283.
8. *Annual report of the Cancer Therapy Evaluation Branch, National Cancer Institute*. Presented at the Second Joint Working Conference, NCI Chemotherapy Program, Annapolis, Maryland, November 3-5, 1971. Washington, D.C., U. S. Govt. Printing Office, 1971.
9. Gehan, E.A.: Early studies of anticancer agents in humans: the question of sample size. *Cancer Chemother Rep, 16*:93, 1962.
10. Sandberg, J. and Goldin, A.: Use of first generation transplants of a slow growing solid tumor for the evaluation of new cancer chemotherapeutic agents. *Cancer Chemother Rep, 55*:233, 1971.
11. Fewer, D., Wilson, C.B., Boldrey, E.B., et al.: The chemotherapy of brain

tumors. Clinical experience with carmustine (BCNU) and vincristine. JAMA 222:549, 1972.

12. Goldin, A. Venditti, J., Humphreys, S., and Mantel, N.: Modification of treatment schedules in the management of advanced mouse leukemia with amethopterin. *J Natl Cancer Inst., 17*: 203, 1956.
13. Skipper, H., Schabel, F., Jr., Mellett, L.B., et al.: Implications of biochemical cytokinetic pharmacologic toxicologic relationships in the design of optimal therapeutic schedules. *Cancer Chemother Rep, 54*: 431, 1970.
14. Howard, A. and Pelc, S.: Synthesis of desoxyribonucleic acid in normal and irradiated cells and its relation to chromosome breakage. *Heredity (Lond), 6*:261, 1953.
15. Skipper, H., Schabel, F., Jr., and Wilcox, W.: Experimental evaluation of potential anticancer agents. XIII. On the criteria and kinetics associated with "curability" of experimental leukemia. *Cancer Chemother Rep, 35*: 1, 1964.
16. Bruce, W.R., and Valeriote, F.A.: Normal and malignant stem cells and chemotherapy. A collection of papers presented at the Twenty-First Annual Symposium on Fundamental Cancer Research, 1967. In *The Proliferation and Spread of Neoplastic Cells*. Baltimore, Williams & Wilkins, 1968, pp. 409-422.
17. Bruce, W.R., and van der Gaag, H.: A quantitative assay for the number of murine lymphoma cells capacble of proliferation *in vivo. Nature (Lond), 199*:79, 1963.
18. Frei, E., III, Bickers, J.N., Hewlett, J.S., et al.: Dose schedules and antitumor studies of Arabinosyl cytosine (NSC 63878). *Cancer Res, 29*:1325, 1969.

CHAPTER TWO

CELL KINETICS OF
MALIGNANT BRAIN TUMORS

Takao Hoshino

INTRODUCTION

ONE FACTOR LEADING TO the recently improved results in the chemotherapy of various human tumors is the clinical application of basic principles learned from kinetic studies of both animal and human tumors.

Early chemotherapists attempted to find the most effective agents without understanding the kinetic characteristics of either normal or cancerous tissues. They simply used the highest doses possible without exceeding the limit of tolerable side effects in normal host tissue. This theory of cancer chemotherapy followed the principles of antibiotic therapy for infectious diseases. The objective of both modes of chemotherapy is the destruction of living organisms or tissues harmful to the host. However, the action of anticancer agents differs considerably from that of antibiotic agents. In antibiotic therapy, drug screening or sensitivity testing is important in determining the appropriate drug and dosage for combating a particular organism. The antibiotic chosen has specific affinity for the microorganism, blocking or destroying essential metabolic pathways either lacking or unimportant in the host. Thus, in most cases, significant therapeutic levels can be reached easily without the threat of serious toxicity to the host.

In contrast to antibiotics, most anticancer agents do not have specific affinity for a given tumor tissue, and the difference between therapeutic and toxic doses is not pronounced. Anticancer agents were developed with the aim of arresting or restricting the proliferation of tissue, and proliferation is common to both normal and neoplastic cells. It was initially believed that malignant cells always proliferated at greater rates than those in normal host

16

tissues, and therefore that a therapeutic advantage could be gained, but recent evidence indicates that often the reverse is true.[1] The proliferation rate of many tumor cells may actually be slower than that of actively proliferating normal cells, such as those in small intestinal epithelium[2] and bone marrow.[3]

In the development of chemotherapeutic protocols, the tendency has been to concentrate largely on the problems of drug selection, dosage, and mode of administration. Only relatively recently has attention been focused on drug scheduling. In the past, most chemotherapeutic trials in both animals and humans consisted of daily doses of an agent continued until the host manifested signs of toxicity. Increased knowledge of proliferation kinetics has indicated that such a standardized approach in drug dose and scheduling was a serious misconception. For example, in many animal tumor systems, oncolytic effects obtained from relatively high doses of alkylating agents spaced at appropriate intervals are much more marked than those from lower doses administered daily on a long-term basis, without any significant increase in host toxicity. It is now recognized that the productive use of phase-specific agents requires optimal periods of effective blood concentrations that must be matched with the cell cycle characteristics and proliferative state of the particular tumor under treatment.

Fundamental information not readily available from any other study source can be gained from kinetic data for use in the scheduling of chemotherapeutic agents. The clinical application of kinetic principles has played a significant role in the improved results which are now being attained in the treatment of several types of leukemia and lymphoma.[4,5] Unfortunately, the study of neoplastic cell kinetics in human leukemias where sampling and cell counting can be done easily and as frequently as required is much simpler in this practical sense than the study of solid tumors. Nevertheless, the growth kinetics of solid tumors must be intensively studied to provide a basis for rational drug scheduling, and it is distinctly possible that some agents that were previously thought to be ineffective in a particular type of tumor could prove useful if kinetic studies indicate that vastly different scheduling protocols are required.

BASIC CONCEPTS OF CELL KINETICS

The neoplastic process can be defined as the unrestricted increase by cell division of the cell population in a host. Proliferation kinetics of a tumor cell population will supply information for analyzing the tumor's growth. The concept of the cell cycle, introduced in 1951,[6] was the initial impetus for the study of tissue growth.

Two classes of cell reproduction are recognized: (1) cell renewal systems, and (2) expanding cell population systems. The cell renewal system is seen in the cellular regeneration of almost every adult tissue, such as bone marrow, epithelium of the small intestine, and skin. No absolute increase in the cell population occurs in these tissues because the birth of a new cell is balanced by the death and loss of another cell. On the other hand, constant population increase is the characteristic feature of the expanding cell population system. This system can be subdivided into: (1) normal expanding tissues, or controlled growth systems, exemplified by embryonal tissue growth, regeneration of the liver after partial hepatectomy, and wound healing in a tissue defect, and (2) uncontrolled systems, as seen in neoplastic growth.

The major difference between these two subdivisions lies in the presence or absence of growth regulation. In normally expanding tissues, a substantial degree of automatic growth regulation exists. When such a tissue reaches an optimal cell population for proper functioning, the majority of its cells become mature and sterile, leaving a small population in the proliferating pool to renew the tissue at a constant maintenance rate. This implies that a cell, once actively proliferating, can become a nonproliferating or resting cell, leading to the conclusion that two types of cells may exist in a tissue, namely those in a proliferating pool and those in a nonproliferating pool.

It was previously thought that all cells in a tumor were proliferating, although at a slow rate. The newer concept is of both a nonproliferating pool tumor cell population and a proliferating pool tumor cell population reproducing at a faster-than-normal rate. The concept of a nonproliferating tumor cell population is now an established fact, but it must be clearly understood that this loss of reproductivity is a transient phenomenon. Such cells can regain their proliferative potential at any time and return to the proliferating pool.

Obligatory cell loss is a feature of all tissue, whether neoplastic or normal. In normal tissue, cells mature, function for a predetermined period, and then die. In neoplastic tissue, however, cell loss — demonstrated by focal or massive necrosis — occurs not as the fate of mature cells but as the result of vascular and/or nutritional crises, ascribed to overcrowding, which affect all cells.

With these concepts in mind, how can each type of growth be characterized from the standpoint of proliferation kinetics? There are four basic parameters by which the growth characteristics of any tumor are expressed, namely: (1) cell cycle time (or cell generation time), (2) tumor doubling time, (3) growth fraction, and (4) cell loss factor. These four parameters are closely interrelated, and the value of any one can be calculated from knowledge of the others.

Cell Cycle Time

Cell cycle time is the time required by a proliferating cell to pass from one mitosis to the next. Not all cells within a population have the same cycle time, and a considerable range of variability exists.[7] The average cell cycle time of a number of cells is used to represent the cycle time in a particular tumor.

Each cell cycle can be divided into four separate stages on the basis of the nuclear desoxyribonucleic acid (DNA) content. The most easily identified stage (by light microscopy) is the M (mitotic) phase, during which the previously duplicated chromosomes are shared between the two daughter cells. These daughter cells then enter the post-mitotic gap (or pre-DNA synthetic) phase — the G1 phase — during which they synthesize ribonucleic acid (RNA), enzymes, and proteins in preparation for the beginning of DNA synthesis. From the G1 phase they move into the DNA synthesis phase — the S phase — in which they replicate DNA. Chromosomal duplication is normally completed by the end of this phase. Following the S phase, another gap (post-synthetic or pre-mitotic) phase — the G2 phase — occurs, during which RNA and proteins are made in preparation for the ensuing mitosis, completing the cycle.

Cells in the G1, S and G2 phase are called intermitotic cells, in contrast to the cells of the mitotic (M) phase. In the G1 phase, the amount of DNA (or number of chromosomes) in the nuclei, normally 2N, increases during the S phase to 4N at the completion of DNA synthesis. It remains at 4N throughout the G2 phase.

Various phases of the cell cycle *in vitro* have been defined from the interpretation of labeled mitosis curves. If exogenous thymidine is presented to a proliferating population of cells, it will be incorporated into the nuclear DNA of those cells which are in S phase at the time of exposure. If the thymidine is labeled with ^{3}H or ^{14}C, nuclei that incorporate thymidine can be identified readily

LABELED MITOSES CURVE OF RAT GLIOMA 9 *IN VIVO*

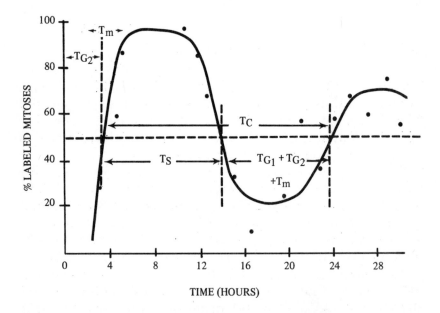

Figure 2-1. Curve of mitotic rat glioma 9 cells labeled after a pulse of ^{3}H-thymidine administered *in vivo*.

by radioautography using conventional techniques. After a pulse or flash labeling of a cell population *in vitro* (brief exposure to radioactive thymidine by injection), by repeated sampling a labeled mitosis curve can be constructed to define the cell cycle time and duration of each phase.[6] Figure 2-1 presents an example of a labeled mitosis curve obtained from a rat glioma model.

A flash label tags all the cells in S phase, and the subsequent progression of this labeled cohort through two successive mitoses is then followed to define the curve. The first labeled mitotic figures will appear after an interval equal to the length of G2 (T_{G2}). The ratio of labeled to total mitoses will approach 1.0 as the tagged cohort proceeds through the M phase. Thus M phase (Tm) can be defined as the time elapsed between the appearance of the first labeled mitosis and the time the index reaches 1.0. Theoretically, S phase will be measured from the length of the first wave. Since this value indicates the longest S phase in this cohort, usually the median duration of S(Ts) can be measured from the midpoints of the ascending and descending limbs of the wave. After an interval equal to Ts + T_{G2} + Tm, all mitoses will be unlabeled, if the cells are synchronized. A second wave of labeled mitoses defines cell cycle time (Tc) and the duration of G1 phase (T_{G1}), which can be obtained from the following formula:

$$T_{G1} = Tc\text{-}(T_{G2} + Tm + Ts) \text{ - - - - -} \quad (1)$$

The proportion of cells labeled after a flash of ^{3}H-thymidine is designated the labeling index (LI); this index indicates the percentage of cells in S phase at any one time and therefore gives a rough indication of the proliferative activity of the tissue. However, while a higher LI indicates greater proliferative activity, equal LI's do not necessarily indicate equal tissue growth. Tissue growth depends not only on the proportion of cells in S phase, but also on the growth fraction of the population (the ratio of proliferating to nonproliferating cells) and on cell loss from the total tumor cell population. In other words, even if two LI's are the same, the doubling times of those tumors may differ dramatically according to the growth fraction and the cell loss of each. In spite of many possible errors in estimating the rate of proliferation by means of the LI alone, it is a useful parameter that yields much kinetic information when combined with other factors such as duration of S phase (Ts).

The Ts can be obtained *in vivo* where multiple sampling is not possible by exposing cells to two different pulses — one with ^{3}H-thymidine, the other with ^{14}C-thymidine — at an interval (t) equivalent to no more than T_{G2}.[8] Because ^{3}H (tritium) is a low energy particle capable of tracking no more than 1μ into an overlying radiographic emulsion, grains of reduced silver will be superimposed directly over the labeled nucleus. The higher energy ^{14}C particles can track for more than 10μ and in autoradiographs of ^{14}C-labeled cells grains will be scattered around, as well as directly over, the nucleus. This difference in labeling characteristics allows separate identification of cells labeled with ^{3}H alone and with ^{14}C plus or minus ^{3}H after staining.

The first flash label (^{3}H) tags the cohort of cells in S phase. At the end of an interval of time (t), a proportion of tagged cells moves into G2 and a proportion of G1 cells moves into S. A second flash label (^{14}C) will then double-label ^{3}H tagged cells still in the S phase and give a ^{14}C tag to G1 cells that have entered S in the interval. One can then calculate the duration of the S phase by the formula:

$$\text{Ts} = \frac{\text{number of cells labeled with } ^{14}\text{C}}{\text{number of cells labeled with } ^3\text{H alone}} \times t \text{ - - -} \quad (2)$$

Since a given number of ^{3}H labeled cells leave the S phase during every interval of t, the time required for all cells in S phase to move into the G2 phase will be expressed by the above equation.*

If all cells are proliferating and are uniformly distributed along

---

*Ts given by this calculation is correct when the influx of cells into S phase equals the efflux of cells from S phase, which is common in cell renewal systems where there is no increase in cell population. However, this value is an overestimate in the expanding cell population system, because the number of cells entering S phase should be more than that of cells leaving the S phase, even though the former will nearly equal the latter with increasing cell loss and lengthening of the G1 phase.[9]

the cell cycle, one can obtain cell cycle time from the following formula:

$$Tc = (Ts/LI) \times 100 - - - - - - \tag{3}$$

(LI = labeling index in percent)

All newly labeled cells will pass into G2 and beyond after a period of time equal to Ts, and their place in the S compartment of the tumor cell population will be occupied by unlabeled cells from the G1 compartment. The cell cycle time (Tc) in this situation is the time required for all the cells to pass through S phase. If nonproliferating cells constitute a fraction of the population, then this value obtained from the above equation does not equal the cell cycle time, but indicates the time required for the production of a number of cells equal to those already present (turnover time). When only one of the two daughter cells enters into another mitotic cycle, this value is also equal to the potential doubling time, which reflects the doubling time free of cell loss (Tp). Such a circumstance could be similar to that of the cell renewal systems where one of the daughter cells moves to the nonproliferating pool on differentiation.

If one assumes that both daughter cells enter into another cell cycle (an event common in neoplastic tissue), the calculated value from the equation will have theoretical significance only and will exceed the Tp of the tumor. A variable conversion coefficient k, which will provide an approximate Tp from this value, has been calculated by Steel.[10]

$$Tp = k \times \frac{Ts}{LI} \times 100 - - - - - - \tag{4}$$

In those cases where the expected doubling time exceeds one-hundred hours, k is close to 0.7. The cell cycle time can also be obtained by determining the median grain index-halving time after a single pulse of ^{3}H-thymidine since, after each cell division, the labeled DNA of the parent cell will theoretically be equally distributed to the two daughter cells.[11]

The same information can be obtained by continuous labeling[12,13] with ³H-thymidine, either by infusion or by multiple pulses separated by an interpulse interval less than Ts. The ratio between the initial LI and its increase per unit time gives Ts; and the interval of time from the first pulse of ³H-thymidine until the ascending LI curve levels out gives Tc. The use of ³H-thymidine combined with Colchicine® or similar chemicals which arrest mitosis at metaphase, has also provided data for determining the duration of the cell cycle and its individual phases.[14] If *in vitro* observation is feasible, Tc may be obtained by using time-lapse cinephotomicrography to follow a cell from one mitosis to another.[13]

In clinical situations where either phase-specific or cycle-specific drugs are to be used, knowledge of the values of the various parameters of the cell cycle which have been described in this section is important. During every course of treatment, one would like to have therapeutic drug levels in contact with the tumor for at least the duration of one complete cell cycle. In this way, the greatest number of susceptible cells will be destroyed.

Growth Fraction

Growth fraction is an index of the relationship of the proliferating cell population to the total tumor cell population. The concept of the possible existence of nonproliferating cells in a tumor cell population was first suggested by Baserga, et al.[15] in 1960; in 1962, Mendelsohn [16] calculated the mathematical definition of this factor and introduced it into population kinetics. Accumulated data on growth fractions have explained part of the discrepancy between growth calculated on the basis of the cell cycle time and growth actually observed in tumor systems. Growth fraction (GF) is expressed in the following formula:

$$GF = \frac{\text{proliferating pool cells}}{\text{total cell population}} \quad - - - - - \quad (5)$$

This formula has little practical value, since the number of cells in the proliferating pool cannot be measured. There is no way to differentiate the nonproliferating pool (G_0) cells from those in G1 phase at any specified time. An estimation of GF could be obtained by continuous labeling of the tumor with ^{3}H-thymidine beyond one cycle time so that all cells in the proliferating pool would pass at least once through S phase and be labeled; those remaining unlabeled would represent the G_0 population. The GF derived in this way might be an overestimate since there can be no guarantee that all the labeled cells will remain proliferating; some may already have moved into the nonproliferating pool.

Presently, there are two other methods of calculating GF. The first is:

Since $\dfrac{\text{cells in S phase}}{\text{cells in S phase}} = 1$, formula (5) can be rewritten:

$$GF = \frac{\text{cells in proliferating pool}}{\text{total cell population}} \quad \text{x} \quad \frac{\text{cells in S phase}}{\text{cells in S phase}}$$

$$= \frac{\text{cells in proliferating pool}}{\text{cells in S phase}} \quad \text{x} \quad \frac{\text{cells in S phase}}{\text{total cell population}}$$

The right bracket represents the LI and the left bracket represents the reciprocal of the so-called theoretical labeling index (TLI), which is the ratio of cells in S phase to cells in proliferating pool. Thus, the growth fraction can be expressed as the ratio of observed LI to TLI:

$$GF = \frac{LI}{TLI} \text{ - - - -} \tag{6}$$

If the cell cycle time of the tumor and the durations of T_{32} and Ts phases are known, the TLI can be calculated from the formula derived by Cleaver[17]:

$$TLI = \frac{Ts}{Tc} \log 2 + \frac{1}{2}\frac{Ts}{Tc} \text{ x } \log 2^2 + \frac{Ts \text{ x } T}{Tc^2} \quad \text{x } \log 2^2 \text{ - - } \tag{7}$$

The second method for calculating the TLI proposed by Mendelsohn[16] is to establish the ratio of labeled to total mitoses several generation times after the pulse of ^{3}H-thymidine (Figure 2-2).

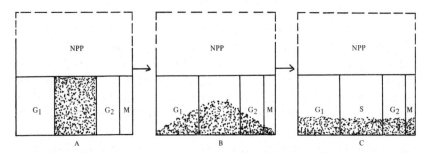

Figure 2-2. (A) Cells in S phase are labeled by a pulse of ^{3}H-thymidine. TLI is the ratio of labeled cells/cells in G$_1$, S, G$_2$, and M phases. (B) After one generation time, cells in the proliferating pool have doubled in number and so have the labeled cells. The ratio of labeled cellsDtotal proliferating cells remains constant. However, overlap of labeled cohort occurs on either side of S phase due to desynchronization. (C) Several generation times later, labeled cells will be distributed evenly throughout the cell cycle and the ratio of labeled mitoses/total mitoses represents labeled cells/cells in proliferating pool, which is the TLI. NPP = cells in nonproliferating pool; G$_1$ = cells in G$_1$ phase; S = cells in S phase; G$_2$ = cells in G$_2$ phase; M = cells in M phase; shaded area = cells labeled by ^{3}H-thymidine.

The GF is an index of the proportion of the tumor that will be susceptible to cell cycle- or phase-specific drugs. It would be injudicious to treat a tumor having a small GF with cycle- or phase-dependent drugs as a first choice, for they could not reduce the tumor size to an extent that would be beneficial to the host. If, after all proliferating cells are destroyed by an effective cycle-specific agent, cells in the unaffected nonproliferating pool remained in a nonproliferating stage, there would be no subsequent increase in tumor size. However, in most malignant solid tumors, including those of the brain, the nonproliferating pool supplies cells to replace those in the proliferating pool that are destroyed by cycle-specific agents.

It is not understood how, when, or in what proportion nonproliferating cells are released into the proliferating pool after a single course of chemotherapy. This is the most difficult problem remaining to be solved but it is evident that such information could be of immense aid in chemotherapy scheduling.

Population Doubling Time and Cell Loss

Population doubling time (Td), commonly termed doubling time, should not be confused with the cell cycle (generation) time (Tc). Doubling time signifies the interval required for the whole cell population to double in number; the value of the Td is the same as the cycle time only when all cells are proliferating (GF = 1) in synchronous phase and there is no cell loss.

As stated earlier, GF is commonly less than 1.0 in many tissues and tumors and so the Td invariably exceeds Tc. Proliferating pool cells must divide several times to double the total population, compensating for the nonproliferating fraction and for cells lost. If one assumes that a proportion of newborn cells constantly moves into the nonproliferating pool, the Td can then be derived by a mathematical equation.

However, the observed doubling time (Td) is usually longer than the calculated time (or potential doubling time, Tp). This discrepancy between the Td and Tp can be attributed to the cell loss factor, as formulated by Steel.[10] Cell loss in a tumor is easily demonstrated by the presence of massive or focal necrosis and exfoliation of cells from the tumor mass. Quantitative estimation of the loss is difficult. To express the magnitude of cell loss, Steel devised the cell loss factor (CLF) as:

$$CLF = 1 - \frac{Tp}{Td} - - - - - \qquad (8)$$

This factor represents the rate of cell loss as a fraction of the rate at which cells are added to the total population by mitosis. Thus, a CLF = 1.0 (or 100%) indicates that cell loss is counter-balanced by cell production, with neither growth nor regression of tumor, i.e., the total cell population remains constant. On the other hand, a cell loss factor of 0 implies exponential growth, and in such a situation, Td is the same as Tp. Although the Tp and the CLF are, in a sense, theoretical values, they allow comparison of the importance of cell loss as a determinant of growth rate among different tumor types. These values are generally dependent on the size as well as the nature of the tumor; increase in tumor size results in greater cell loss and longer doubling time.

Although these parameters have little relevance to therapeutic scheduling, they are significant in clinical prognosis. Additionally, any change in doubling time or in cell loss factor is helpful in evaluating the effects of chemotherapy.

CELL RENEWAL VS. NEOPLASTIC GROWTH

An imperative consideration in the chemotherapy of malignant tumors is a given agent's side effects. Virtually all anticancer drugs exert their effects by interfering with metabolic processes that are common to both tumor cells and all proliferating tissues although the rate of proliferation may be different for tumor cells and the various types of regenerating tissue within the same host.

Figure 2-3, modified from Cleaver,[9] illustrates a comprehensive model of the adult cell renewal system. Two proliferating compartments are proposed in this model; (1) a stem cell compartment, which is self-maintaining and proliferates at a very slow rate, and (2) a second proliferating compartment, which accelerates the proliferation rate of daughter cells originating in the stem cell compartment and boosts the total number of cells reaching maturation. Since the cells in this latter compartment proliferate

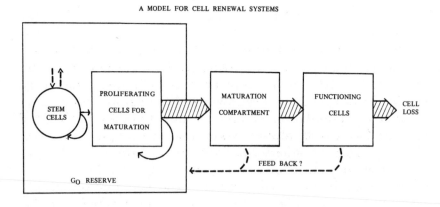

Figure 2-3. Conceptual model of cell renewal system. See explanation in text. (Modified from Cleaver,[9] p. 191.)

more rapidly than the stem cells, the kinetics of the cell renewal system will depend on the division rate of these daughter cells.[18] Once a cell has reached maturation, it ceases to proliferate; the cell then prepares enzymes and proteins for its assigned role in the functioning tissue. The key to the cell renewal system is the maintenance of an equilibrium of the total cell population, that is, the balancing of cell loss by equal cell generation from the proliferating compartments.

This conceptual model has not been completely proven, but it does satisfy several experimental observations, such as the lag in the onset of side-effects or the recovery time of a tissue system after chemotherapy. For example, bone marrow intoxication and recovery after antimetabolite therapy can be explained by postulating that more stem cells escape from the effects of chemotherapy because of their slow proliferative activity, compared to the more marked involvement of the daughter cells in the proliferating compartments. The series of events which would occur after chemotherapy is as follows: Tissue functioning remains normal until unaffected mature and functioning cells become senescent and die. This period corresponds to the time lag before side-effects appear. Toxicity becomes manifest with a reduction in the number of mature cells. The toxic effects of the chemotherapeutic agent prevent the cells in the second proliferative compartment from entering the maturation compartment. The stem cells, being minimally affected by the drug, then start feeding cells to the proliferating compartment, and consequently the deficiency in functioning cells will be corrected gradually. Severe degrees of toxicity, such as in bone marrow, result either from an extreme loss in the functioning cell compartment, or alternately, from a failure of the stem cell compartment to return a sufficient number of cells to the proliferative compartments and thus replenish the tissue. (Fig. 2-4).

The question arises: Do neoplasms contain a counterpart to stem cells in normal tissue? There is evidence suggesting the existence of cells in such a compartment, termed by some the clonogenic or colony-forming cells.[19] These cells cannot be differentiated from other proliferating tumor cells by microscopic or biochemical means, but their presence has been indirectly proven

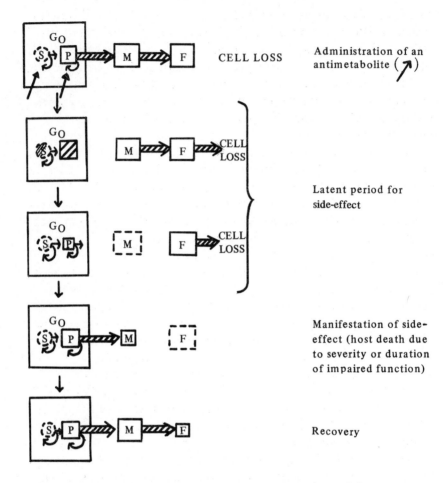

Figure 2-4. Conceptual model of possible mechanism of bone marrow intoxication and recovery after antimetabolite therapy. Refer to the cell renewal model in Figure 2-3. $G_0 = G_0$ (nonproliferating) cell reserve; S = stem cell compartment; P = proliferating cells for maturation; M = maturation compartment; F = functioning cells. Details in text.

by the ability of such cells when isolated to give rise to separate tumors.

It was stated earlier in this chapter that, from the kinetic point of view, uncontrolled growth was the basic difference between neoplastic and normal tissue. More specifically, using tumor models, three mechanisms have been substantiated to explain this uncontrolled growth. They are: (1) shortening of the length of the cell cycle, (2) reduction of cell loss, and (3) increase of the recycling cell population, either by the movement of cells from G_0 to $G1$ compartment or by blocking of the pathway to nondividing compartments.

A shortening of the cell cycle time plays a definite role in the rate of tumor growth in some experimental systems, and it seems proportionate to the degree of tumor malignancy.[20] On the other hand, there is much evidence that the cell cycle time of certain tumors is far longer than that of the tissue from which the tumor originated.[1] The reduction of cell loss is significant in the development of certain animal tumors, but for human[21,22] tumors the relative roles of cell loss and prolongation of the cell life span have not been fully documented. Increase in the proliferative cell

A TUMOR MODEL

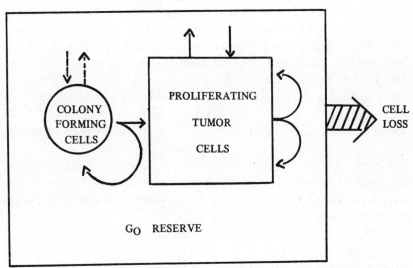

Figure 2-5. Conceptual model of possible mechanism of tumor growth. Compare this model with normal cell renewal system in Figure 2-3. Chemotherapy should be aimed at colony-forming cells.

population by blocking of the pathway towards maturation may play an important role in neoplastic alteration of tissue. In fact, all of the above factors probably have a role in tumor cell population kinetics.

Although many of these concepts remain theoretical, they have led to useful lines of chemotherapeutic investigation (Fig. 2-5). From the above discussion, it is obvious that in any tumor only the stem or colony-forming cells need to be destroyed. Investigations aimed at identifying these cells and finding their metabolic properties are important and should be pursued.

CURRENT INFORMATION ON
BRAIN TUMOR PROLIFERATION

In terms of its kinetic characteristics, the brain is one of the most unusual organs of the body, since it is known that neurons do not undergo mitotic division past a period shortly after birth. The glial cells, making up the supportive tissue in the brain, continue to proliferate as demonstrated by the phenomenon of gliosis,[23] but so far there is no evidence that they do so at more than a minimal rate. There are several reports suggesting that a low level of mitotic activity is continually present in the glial population within the adult rat brain.[24,25] This experimental work indicates that the production of new cells by very slow proliferative activity is enough to balance glial cell loss, but the rate is too low for measurement of cell cycle time by current methods.

Kinetic data on normal adult human brain is not available, but incidental examination of unaffected portions of brain in brain tumor patients to whom ³H-thymidine has been administered has revealed almost no labeled cells, suggesting very low regenerative activity. Nevertheless, there may be limited areas of the brain where more active proliferation does take place, similar to the subependymal layer of adult rat ventricles, although no intensive study has been carried out in man. The kinetic state of normal brain tissue clearly contrasts with that of brain tumors, in which the extent of the proliferating population can readily be appreciated. The boundaries imposed by ethical considerations and the heterogeneity of solid tumors in man preclude the direct application of routine kinetic analytic methods to clinical material.

Techniques requiring multiple, long-term sampling of specimens cannot be applied to human brain tumors. Thus, data that may be useful in predicting proliferative activity must be obtained from material in a single biopsy after suitable ³H-thymidine administration.

The first *in vivo* study of a human glioblastoma was carried out by Johnson, et al. in 1960.[26] They administered multiple doses of ³H-thymidine, and since their method of administration was neither a single pulse nor continuous labeling, it is difficult to interpret the LI obtained. Assuming the duration of S phase to be six hours, they calculated the generation time of a glioblastoma to be six to eight weeks. Chigasaki[27] studied the *in vitro* uptake of ³H-thymidine by biopsy specimens of a glioblastoma, an astrocytoma, and an oligodendroglioma, obtaining LI's of 0.94, 0.44, and 0.33 percent respectively. He utilized the same formula as Johnson for calculating the generation time of each tumor, but chose to assume seven hours for the S phase. He estimated the generation time of the glioblastoma to be twenty-two to thirty-one days, and those of the astrocytoma and the oligodendroglioma to be forty-five to sixty and sixty to ninety days respectively. Both papers neglected the possible role of cell loss and the factor of the nonproliferating compartment in the process of calculation, and confused generation time with doubling time. In spite of this difference in terminology, their results coincided fairly well with the clinical behavior of each tumor.

A few years later, Kury and Carter[28] examined the *in vitro* LI of several gliomas using a method almost identical to Chigasaki's, and reported that two glioblastomas had LI's of 3.6 percent and 6.0 percent and five astrocytomas (grade two to three) had labeling indices of 2 percent, 2 percent, 2.6 percent, 5.5 percent and 7.4 percent, all considerably higher than those reported by Johnson, et al. and Chigasaki. They estimated generation times (approximately equal to Tp) of glioblastomas and malignant astrocytomas to be three to five days and two to ten days respectively, assuming an S phase of six hours. From this, they concluded that the LI increased as the grade of malignancy increased, although the calculated generation time of each tumor is far from that reported by former authors.

Fukuma, et al.,[29] using local injection of ³H-thymidine into glioma tissue at the time of craniotomy, reported a LI for astrocytomas without anaplasia of 1.5 percent to 4.6 percent, for anaplastic astrocytomas and glioblastomas of 2.6 percent to 11.0 percent, and for a medulloblastoma and an ependymoglioblastoma in infants, 8.1 percent and 3.3 percent respectively. They applied an S phase of twenty-four hours for the calculation of generation time of the medulloblastoma and the ependymoblastoma using the formula of Johnson, et al. and obtained 8.5 to 12.3 days and 21 to 30.3 days respectively.

In all of these studies only the LI was experimentally determined. The duration of S phase was assumed to expand their arguments. Hence the experimental determination of the S phase becomes critical in order to confirm their conclusions.

Tym[30] introduced the stathmokinetic method, adding the use of vinblastine sulfate to the flash labeling technique. Using only one glioblastoma patient, he obtained a LI of 1.6 percent and calculated a G2 phase of five hours, an S phase of eight hours, and a cell cycle time of 125 hours (5.4 days) to 242 hours (10 days).

The author's own recent studies [31] revealed that LI's varied widely between individual tumors and between different areas from the same tumor; for example, the LI within necrotic areas was nearly zero, while the LI within the viable part of the same tumor might approach 20 percent. However, the LI's correlated within similar histologic areas of different tumors of the same grade. By means of double radioautography technique, he also estimated the duration of S phase in each tumor and calculated turnover time.

Table 2-I summarizes these kinetic parameters on twelve brain tumors. Labeling indices are expressed in percents. The range indicates the minimum and the maximum LI for the various tumor types, calculated by examining groups of approximately 1,000 cells in different areas of each tumor. By this method, glioblastoma multiforme had an average LI of 5 percent to 10 percent and astrocytoma of 1 percent or less. The LI of anaplastic astrocytomas fell between that of well-differentiated astrocytomas and that of glioblastomas, depending on the degree of anaplasia of different tumor areas. For example, an area containing well-differentiated astrocytes, with or without microcysts, showed a LI

close to that of astrocytomas, whereas an area containing anaplastic astrocytes with neoplastic vascular changes showed a LI
resembling similar areas within glioblastomas. A pilocytic area
in a glioblastoma multiforme showed a far higher LI than that of
otherwise identical pilocytic areas within astrocytomas. This suggests that the pilocytic astrocytes found in glioblastomas are quite
different biologically from pilocytic astrocytes in astrocytomas in
spite of morphological similarities, and implies a different on-
cological origin of these two tumors, not withstanding a more or
less similar malignant prognosis. In contrast to the variability of
the LI in different tumors, the duration of S phase remained in the
seven to ten hour range regardless of tumor type and degree of
malignancy. Many factors may influence the duration of S phase
in vivo, but among neoplastic astrocytes the data seem to exclude
varying grades of biologic malignancy.

The author's results on S phase duration are quite close to those
obtained by Tym and considerably shorter than those found in
other tumor types such as leukemias,[32,33] and epitheliomas,[34,35]
the range of which is from ten to twenty hours. This difference in
S phase length between brain tumors and other tumor types could
possibly be ascribed to variability in procedural technique. The
turnover time of brain tumors, derived from the LI and S phase
using formula (3), is shorter in malignant gliomas (on the order of
a few days to a week) and longer in astrocytomas (two months).

The Tp obtained by multiplying the turnover time by the conversion factor (k = 0.7, discussed earlier in this chapter[10]), indicates
that malignant gliomas, including glioblastomas, would double
their size in less than five days excluding cell loss. Since the LI and
the duration of S phase were measured only in viable parts of each
tumor, the true LI should be lower in proportion to the ratio of
viable to total tumor cell population. For example, if one assumes
that one-third of the tumor mass is made up of necrotic cells, the
true LI for the whole tumor is reduced by a factor of 2/3, yielding a
longer Tp by a factor of 3/2. Clinically, it is well known that
glioblastomas and malignant astrocytomas grow quickly. However, at their symptomatic size (i.e., 50 to 100 gm), it is impossible
to accept that these tumors double their size every week or so, even
taking the above modifications into consideration. To explain

Brain Tumor Chemotherapy

TABLE 2-I

KINETIC PARAMETERS IN BRAIN TUMORS*

CASE	PATHOLOGY	LI	T_s	BR	T_{over}
W.S.	glioblastoma	5.9	5 hrs.	1.28	79 hrs.
J.T.	glioblastoma	11.4	7	1.71	59
C.P.	glioblastoma	8.1	-	-	-
F.C.	glioblastoma	5.5	10	0.59	191
L.M.	glioblastoma	4.4	9	0.49	203
E.M.	malignant astrocytoma	5.4	11	0.51	198
L.S.	malignant astrocytoma	8.2	13	0.65	156
R.E.	malignant astrocytoma	2.3	7	0.33	307
H.S.	astrocytoma	1.0	-	-	-
M.M.	astrocytoma	0.8	10	0.09	1154
H.J.	metastatic	6.3	7	0.92	108
W.S.	metastatic	13.6	-	-	-

LI = labeling index
T_s = duration of S phase
BR = Birth Rate = Number of new cells/100 cells/hour
T_{over} = Turnover Time = 100 cells/BR

*Modified from Hoshino, T. and Wilson, C. B.: "Principles of Tumor Cell Population Kinetics and their Application to Brain Tumors: A Review" *J Neurosurg, 42*:123-131, 1975.

this discrepancy, one must assume extensive cell loss within the tumor. A tentative calculation, assuming a Tp of a week and a Td of six weeks, gives a CLF of 0.85 (or 85%), which, surprisingly, is not high when compared to those estimated for other tumors, e.g. head and neck, 95 percent,[21] melanomas, 70 percent.[34]

Astrocytomas are characterized by a lower LI, a longer turnover time, and almost the same S period as other brain tumors. Presumably, this indicates that the population of an astrocytoma increases at a slower rate. Histological studies of astrocytomas show a fairly homogeneous distribution of well-differentiated astrocytes and moderate vascularity without prominent perivascular proliferation or endothelial thickening. Some astrocytomas lack the dense cellularity and compactness characteristic of glioblastomas, which suggests that crowding of cells does not account for the inhibition of cell proliferation. On the basis of their histological patterns, astrocytoma cells do not appear to suffer from a lack of essential substrates, seemingly one of the main factors limiting growth of malignant gliomas and other rapidly growing tumors. Cell loss in astrocytomas should be less than that of malignant gliomas, as reflected by the absence of massive necrosis. The main cause of the existing cell loss will be abortive mitosis and cell death by aging or degeneration. Thus, the observed LI in this kind of tumor is close to the true LI.

These observations may indicate that cells in well-differentiated astrocytomas either have a very long cell cycle time or reside mostly in the nonproliferating pool. A gradual increase in mass is maintained at the same steady rate in most well-differentiated astrocytomas, independent of their size, and this may reflect a biological characteristic ensuring a very low GF throughout the span of tumor growth. The fact that many patients with well-differentiated astrocytomas survive for a number of years after incomplete surgical tumor excision could indicate that there is an insignificant movement of nonproliferating pool cells into the very small proliferating pool, and this may be a characteristic of this tumor type. Surgical removal of this kind of tumor, even if incomplete, and although giving the residual tumor space in which to expand, effectively reduces the cells in the proliferating pool.

Clinical experience demonstrates that this situation is not true of malignant gliomas, which have a higher GF and a more frequent transition of nonproliferating cells into the proliferating pool. Growth in malignant gliomas seems to be depressed by crowding, and partial removal of the tumor will stimulate nonproliferating cells to move into the proliferating pool, causing rapid repopulation of the tumor. Thus, partial surgical removal will not accomplish a significant reduction in the proliferating population; in fact, shortly after excision, the growth fraction becomes higher, and as a corollary, the tumor will be susceptible to cycle- or phase-specific drugs.

The object, therefore, must be to kill not only the proliferating cells in the residual mass, but also to attack the nonproliferating cells retaining the capacity to enter the proliferating pool. Large solid tumors such as glioblastomas will respond less to cycle-specific or phase-specific anticancer drugs because (1) proliferating pool cells, which are the fraction attacked by these drugs, are relatively few, and (2) regrowth from remaining cells in the nonproliferating pool soon replaces the population eliminated by chemotherapy. The author's studies indicate a GF of 30 percent in a viable area of a glioblastoma.[36,37] This value implies that 30 percent of viable cells in a glioblastoma could be killed by cycle-specific drugs or prolonged administration of phase-specific drugs, but this amounts to a reduction of tumor diameter around 10 percent.

Careful investigation as to when and how the transition of cells from the nonproliferating to the proliferating pool occurs may provide clues for the improved therapeutic application of oncolytic agents. However, progress in this regard will be retarded until more information is obtained about the biological characteristics of astrocytic tumors, not only from the viewpoint of proliferation kinetics but also at the level of molecular and subcellular mechanisms.

REFERENCES

1. Post, J., and Hoffman, J.: In vivo replication of normal and tumor cells: relation to cancer chemotherapy. In *Human Tumor Cell Kinetics,*

National Cancer Institute Monograph 30, Bethesda, 1969, pp. 209-224.
2. Lipkin, M.: Cell proliferation in the gastrointestinal tract of man. *Fed Proc, 24*:10, 1965.
3. Blackett, N.M.: The proliferation and maturation of hemopoietic cells. In Baserga, R. (Ed.): *The Cell Cycle and Cancer.* New York, Dekker, 1971, pp. 27-53.
4. Schabel, F.M., Jr.: In vivo leukemic cell kinetics and "curability" in experimental systems. In *The Proliferation and Spread of Neoplastic Cells,* a collection of papers presented at the Twenty-First Annual Symposium on Fundamental Cancer Research, 1967. Baltimore, Williams & Wilkins, 1968, pp. 379-408.
5. Freireich, E.J., Henderson, E.S., Karon, M.R., and Frei, E., III: The treatment of acute leukemia considered with respect to cell population kinetics. In *The Proliferation and Spread of Neoplastic Cells,* A collection of papers presented at the Twenty-First Annual Symposium on Fundamental Cancer Research, 1967. Baltimore, Williams & Wilkins, 1968, pp. 441-452.
6. Howard, A., and Pelc, S.R.: Synthesis of desoxyribonucleic acid in normal and irradiated cells and its relation to chromosome breakage. *Heredity (Lond), 6*:261, 1953.
7. Barrett, J.C.: A mathematical model of the mitotic cycle and its application to the interpretation of percentage labeled mitoses data. *J Natl Cancer Inst, 37*:443, 1966.
8. Wimber, D.E., and Quastler, H.: A C^{14} and ^{3}H-thymidine double labeling technique in the study of cell proliferation in tradescantia root tips. *Exp Cell Res, 30*:8, 1963.
9. Cleaver, J.E.: Population kinetics in animal tissue. In *Thymidine Metabolism and Cell Kinetics,* Amsterdam, North Holland Publishing Co., 1967, pp. 184-234.
10. Steel, G.G.: Cell loss from experimental tumors. *Cell Tissue Kinet, 1*:193, 1968.
11. Cronkite, E.P., Bond, V.P., Fliedner, T.M. and Killman, S.A.: In *Hematopoiesis.* Wolsten Holms and O'Connor, (Eds.) London, Churchill, 1960, pp. 70-98.
12. Robinson, S.H., Brecher, G., Lourie, I.S., and Haley, J.E.: Leukocyte labeling in rats during and after continuous infusion of tritiated thymidine: implications for lymphocyte longevity and DNA reutilization. *Blood, 26*:281, 1965.
13. Sisken, J.E.: Methods for measuring the length of the mitotic cycle and the timing of DNA synthesis for mammalian cells in culture. In Prescott, D.M. (Ed.): *Methods in Cell Physiology.* New York, Acad Pr, 1964, pp. 387-401.
14. Puck, T.T., and Steffen, J.:Life cycle analysis of mammalian cells. I. A method of localizing metabolic events within the life cycle, and its application to the action of colcemide and sublethal doses of

x-irradiation. *Biophys J, 3*:379, 1963.

15. Baserga, R., Kisieleski, W.E., and Halvorsen, K.: A study on the establishment and growth of tumor metastases with tritiated thymidine. *Cancer Res, 20*:910, 1960.

16. Mendelsohn, M.L.: Autoradiographic analysis of cell proliferation in spontaneous breast cancer of C³H mouse. III. The growth fraction. *J Natl Cancer Inst, 28*:1015, 1962.

17. Cleaver, J.E.: The relationship between the duration of the S phase and the fraction of cells which incorporate ³H-thymidine during exponential growth. *Exp Cell Res, 39*:697, 1965.

18. Bond, V.P., Fliedner, T.M., and Archambeau, J.O.: *Mammalian Radiation Lethality. A Disturbance In Cellular Kinetics.* New York, Acad Pr, 1965.

19. Bruce, W.R., and Van der Gaag, H.: A quantitative assay for the number of murine lymphoma cells capable of proliferation in vivo. *Nature (Lond), 199*:79, 1963.

20. Sasaki, T., Morris, H.P., and Baserga, R.: The cell cycles of three transplantable Morris hepatomas. *Cancer Res, 30*:788, 1970.

21. Refsum, S.B., and Berdal, P.: Cell loss in malignant tumours in man. *Eur J Cancer, 3*:235, 1967.

22. Iversen, O.H.: Kinetics of cellular proliferation and cell loss in human carcinomas. A discussion of methods available for in vivo studies. *Eur J Cancer, 3*:389, 1967.

23. Cavanagh, J.B.: The proliferation of astrocytes around a needle wound in the rat brain. *J Anat, 106*:471, 1970.

24. Hommes, O. R., and Leblond, C.P.: Mitotic division of neuroglia in the normal adult rat. *J Comp Neurol, 129*:269, 1967.

25. Lewis, P.D.: The fate of the subependymal cell in the adult rat brain, with a note on the origin of microglia. *Brain, 91*:721, 1968.

26. Johnson, H.A., Haymaker, W.E., Rubini, J.R., et al.: A radioautographic study of a human brain and glioblastoma multiforme after the in vivo uptake of tritiated thymidine. *Cancer, 13*:636, 1960.

27. Chigasaki, H.: Studies on the DNA synthesis function of glial cells by means of ³H-thymidine microradioautography. *Brain Nerve (Tokyo), 15*:767, 1963, (Jap).

28. Kury, G., and Carter, H.W.: Autoradiographic study of human nervous system tumors. *Arch Pathol, 80*:38, 1965.

29. Fukuma, S., Taketoma, S., Ueda, S., et al.: Autoradiographic studies of the growth of brain tumors using local labeling with ³H-thymidine in vivo. *Brain Nerve (Tokyo), 21*:1029, 1969.

30. Tym, R.: Distribution of cell doubling times in in vivo human cerebral tumors. *Surg Forum, 20*:445, 1969.

31. Hoshino, T., Barker, M., Wilson, C.B., et al.: Cell kinetics of human gliomas. *J Neurosurg, 37*:15, 1972.

32. Mauer, A.M., and Fisher, V.: In vivo study of cell kinetics in acute leukemia. *Nature (Lond), 197*:574, 1963.

33. Killmann, S.A., Cronkite, E.P., Fliedner, T.M., and Bond, V.P.: Cell proliferation in multiple myeloma studied with tritiated thymidine in vivo. *Lab Invest, 11*:845, 1962.
34. Shirakawa, S., Luce, J.K., Tannock, I., and Frei, E., III.: Cell proliferation in human melanoma. *J Clin Invest, 49*:1188, 1970.
35. Frindel, E., Malaise, E., and Tubiana, M.: Cell proliferation kinetics in five human solid tumors. *Cancer, 22*:611, 1968.
36. Hoshino, T., and Wilson, C.B.: Principles of tumor cell population kinetics and their application to brain tumors: A review. *J Neurosurg, 42*:123-131, 1975.
37. Hoshino, T., Wilson, C. B., Rosenblum, M. L. and Barker, M.: Chemotherapeutic implications of growth fraction and cell cycle time in glioblastomas. *J. Neurosurg, 43*:127-135, 1975.

CHAPTER **THREE**

PHARMACOLOGICAL CONSIDERATIONS IN BRAIN TUMOR CHEMOTHERAPY*

VICTOR A. LEVIN AND CHARLES B. WILSON

WHEN DESIGNING ANY program of antitumor chemotherapy, the physician must insure that sufficient amounts of the drug or its active principles reach the tumor cells yet avoid untoward systemic toxicity. Thus he will need to consider such factors as molecular size and configuration, lipid solubility, ionization, metabolism, and biotransformation of any chemotherapeutic agent used in the program and how these factors affect drug absorption and delivery to normal brain and tumor. On the basis of these considerations he can then choose the most appropriate drug and route of administration.

GENERAL CONSIDERATIONS

Blood-Brain and CSF Exchange

The interface between blood and brain is unique in human anatomy. Unlike capillaries elsewhere in the body, the endothelial cells of the brain are held tightly together by "welds" between adjacent plasma membranes, called zonulae occludens, which can be observed by electron microscopy.[1] These tight interendothelial junctions appear to be the "barrier" sites for blood-brain exchange of proteins and other large molecular weight substances. They are found in all brain capillaries except a few areas such as the tuber cinereum and area postrema (which have tight junctions between adjoining ependymal cells) and the choroid plexi (where tight junctions occur between adjoining epithelial cells).

*Supported in part by NIH grant CA-13525.

42

Brain capillaries exclude molecules greater than 5 to 7 Å in radius.[2] This is particularly pertinent to water-soluble molecules.[3] In Table 3-I it is evident that creatinine (113 MW) crosses brain capillaries, whereas mannitol (180 MW) does not[4]; somewhere in between is the upper limit of brain capillary permeability.

Figure 3-1 depicts current thinking on blood-brain-cerebrospinal fluid exchange of molecules. The pericapillary space is a small (2 to 4% of brain volume) closed compartment which rapidly equilibrates with blood; it is an anatomic enigma that may have little physiological significance.[5] The extracellular space (ECS) is a compartment representing approximately 16 to 20 percent of brain volume, constant in size in most mammalian species,[6] and probably separate from the glia.[1,4,5] evidence suggests that the ECS is an open-ended compartment in series between plasma and the intracellular space (ICS) and between the intracellular space and the cerebrospinal fluid (CSF).[5]

In animal experiments, diffusion profiles and coefficients have been obtained for molecules that enter cells and cross capillaries, and these have been compared to molecules that do not. Under normal conditions, extracellular transport of water-soluble molecules is by diffusion,[4,6] and there is little restriction of molecular exchange between the ECS and the CSF, for example at the ependyma and the arachnoid. Only for small, nonionized molecules

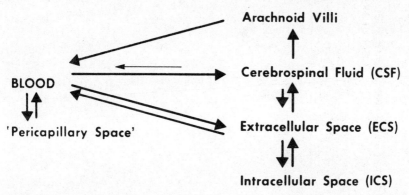

Figure 3-1. Schematic representation of movement of drug molecules between blood and various area in normal brain.

TABLE 3-I

RELATIONSHIP OF MOLECULAR WEIGHT, DIFFUSION COEFFICIENT, DISTRIBUTION SPACE
CELLULAR ENTRY, AND CAPILLARY PERMEABILITY[1]

SUBSTANCE	MW	APP D/AGAR D	DISTRIBUTION SPACE %	INTRACELLULAR ENTRY	TRANSCAPILLARY EXCHANGE
Inulin	5,000	.42	19	-	-
Sucrose	342	.41	19	-	-
PAH	194	.28	25	+	-
Mannitol	184	.24	31	+	-
Fructose	180	.09	54	++	+
Creatine	113	.11	69	++	+
Urea	60	.11	47	++	++
³HOH	18	-	4	++	++

(e.g., urea, antipyrine, ethylene glycol) is resistance sufficiently high to impede exchange, and even in these cases the net effect is negligible.

Table 3-I shows the relationship for various substances of: the molecular weight; the diffusion coefficient in brain (apparent D) over the free-water diffusion coefficient in 2 percent agar gel (agar D); the distribution space (distribution space is defined as percent volume distribution of an isotope in 1 g of tissue); and the ability of the molecule to cross capillaries and/or enter cells. For inulin and sucrose, the 40 percent slower diffusion rate in apparent D than in free water or agar D is thought to be due to the intercellular tortuosity and increased path length that the diffusing molecules follow in the extracellular space.[4] Reading from top to bottom on the table, the apparent D/agar D decrease reflects molecule loss from the extracellular space by passive entry into cells and passive transport across capillaries. From these studies it appears that nonionized water-soluble molecules smaller than 194 MW enter brain cells and that molecules of approximately 140 MW cross brain capillaries. One would anticipate that drugs of approximately 130 MW or less (e.g., 5-FU, hydroxyurea) would readily cross even normal brain capillaries.

For lipid-soluble molecules, the higher the lipid-water partition coefficient of a drug, the greater the rate of penetration into brain.[7,8] However, excess lipid solubility can preclude water solubility in plasma required for optimal transcapillary exchange. In addition, lipid solubility alone does not assure blood-brain passage; as with water-soluble molecules, upper molecular weight and structural limitations exist, although some lipid-soluble molecules of 450 MW enter brain.

At physiologic pH many molecules form weak organic acids or bases, which are prevented from crossing the blood-brain barrier by virtue of their ionization. In such cases, the amount of drug available to cells will depend on the pKa of the drug and the size of the nonionized fraction. For example, Methotrexate (MTX), a commonly used chemotherapeutic agent, is less than 3 percent nonionized at pH 7.3; only this small nonionized fraction can actually enter brain tumor cells.[9]

If the active form of a drug is systemically transformed into an ionized metabolite, the metabolite's penetration of the blood-brain barrier and cell membranes is governed by the rules already given. If the drug is metabolized after entering cells, (e.g., 5-FU, cyclocytidine), ionization of the parent compound occurs intracellularly, usually through phosphorylation.

One way that the brain "disposes" of cellular metabolites provides insight into normal brain-ECS-CSF exchange. Unidirectional ICS→ECS→CSF transport functions as a "sink" for products of brain metabolism[8,10]; this appears to occur by diffusion from ICS→ECS→CSF and by bulk flow from CSF→sagittal sinus blood.[10,11] The entry of water-soluble drugs into the brain from the CSF can be predicted from the drug's diffusion coefficient and molecular weight and configuration (the relationship is actually more closely correlated with atomic radius, but

TABLE 3-II

"GEOMETRY" OF AN INTRACEREBRAL TUMOR

	Central	Growing Edge (BAT)	Brain
Tumor cells (%)	95	15	0
Growth fraction	low	high	--
"Extracellular" or Inulin space (%)	31-32	12-?*	3.5-4.0†
Vital dye (trypan blue) staining	+++	+	0
Blood flow	↑or↓	↓	normal
Capillary permeability	↑	↓	normal
Water content	↑↑	↑	normal
Sodium content	↑↑	↑	normal

*Nonequilibrium value at 6 hr.

†By ventricular perfusion the ECS is 16-29%.

molecular weight proves to be a good approximation).

Blood-Brain Tumor Exchange

Table 3-II is derived from previous experimental studies in intracerebral mouse and rat tumors as well as human tumors. It summarizes certain characteristics of a tumor located within the brain.

The central areas of most tumors studied have had a low growth fraction of 5 to 15 percent, with a variable degree of necrosis. Tumor adjacent to the tumor-brain interface invariably has a higher growth fraction (40 to 50%), reflecting the fact that the growth fraction increases radially from the center to the periphery of the main tumor mass.[13] In the author's studies, use of selected sections has usually defined the number of neoplastic cells in the brain directly adjacent to tumor, as 10 to 15 percent infiltrating tumor cells. Ordinarily one cannot observe differences in capillary structure such as hyperplasia, abnormal endothelialization, or widespread nuclear abnormalities in brain adjacent to tumor. The water content is highest in the tumor and only slightly above normal in brain adjacent to tumors[15]; the extracellular space, determined by inulin (blood side-determination), is nearly twice as large in tumor as in normal brain,[9,14] and intermediate in the brain adjacent to tumor.

In addition, although both increased and decreased blood flow have been observed in brain adjacent to tumor, more frequently blood flow is decreased 20 to 30 percent.[15,16] In the author's laboratories direct measurements of brain adjacent to tumor using twenty-second ^{3}HOH tissue-uptake levels in intracerebral rat sarcoma 9L demonstrated similar extraction ratios in brain, tumor, and brain adjacent to tumor, which raises yet other questions concerning blood flow, capillary permeability, and extraction of ^{3}HOH.[17]

Two observations concerning the blood-brain tumor barrier and the tumor cell barrier are supported by radiological, pathological, and physiological studies. Generally, in gliomatous and most metastatic tumors, the more malignant the tumor, the more permeable its capillaries (with some possible exceptions such as meningiomas and schwannomas); and the more malignant (anaplastic, undifferentiated, etc.) the cell type, the more permeable the tumor cells. More highly malignant tumors tend to be more positive on radionuclide brain scintiscans.[18,19] The vessels of more malignant tumors exhibit proportionately more endothelial hyperplasia, fewer interendothelial tight junctions, more endothelial perforations, and more edema.[7,20,24] Experiments have shown that in low and middle grade murine gliomas the blood-brain barrier allows a molecule as large as [13C]inulin (> 5000 MW) unrestricted entry into the extracellular space, [9,14,25] while highly malignant, viral-induced fibrosarcomas in dogs are highly permeable even to $Tc^{99}m$ human serum albumin (HSA; > 100,000 MW).[26] At the cellular lzvel, the low and middle grade glioma cells behave more like normal brain cells in excluding p-aminohippurate (PAH; 194 MW) reasonably well, although they may allow more rapid entry of mannitol (184 MW) and urea (60 MW).[25] However, in the more malignant leptomeningeal fibrosarcoma, the cell barrier is permeable even to inulin. Figure 3-2 depicts the uptake of some standard molecules into the murine glioma, demonstrating the direct relationship of entry rate and distribution to molecular size. In normal brain,

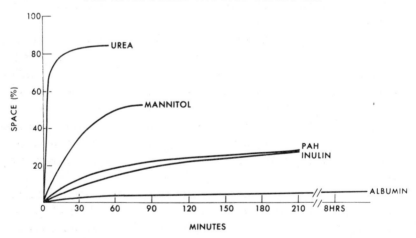

Figure 3-2. Uptake curves demonstrating the direct relationship of molecular weight to rate and degree of penetration of some standard molecules into the intracerebral murine glioma.

mannitol, PAH, and inulin distribute from blood in a 2 to 4 percent space, and albumin in a 1 to 4 percent space.[14,25] More studies are required to further document and expand these observations, but certain conclusions seem justified.

Another characteristic of brain tumors is peritumoral edema. In most cases the extracellular edema and increased capillary permeability within the tumor appear to be responsible for edema fluid in the extracellular space of surrounding brain (particularly in white matter). However, in some very small metastatic tumors a disproportionate amount of hemispheral swelling suggests additional humoral factors. The explanation for the latter phenomenon is unknown.

Using human choriocarcinoma implanted in the cerebrum of the rhesus monkey, the author found that $Tc^{99}m$-HSA and ^{14}C-inulin moved into surrounding brain from the tumor primarily by diffusion.[27] Complementary experiments in rats (implanted intracerebrally with Walker 256 carcinosarcomas and 9L sarcomas induced with methyl nitrosourea) have shown that the immediate peritumoral brain did not have the increased capillary permeability found in tumors, but actually had a 40 percent reduction in capillary permeability to ^{24}Na and ^{14}C-urea when compared to normal brain.[17] These experiments also showed that as early as six minutes after isotope injection, much of the isotope found in the brain adjacent to tumor originated from the tumor. From these experiments it was concluded that the decrease in capillary permeability was not secondary to a reduction in capillary surface area in the brain adjacent to tumor.

The above studies imply that polar drugs will enter the regions of infiltrative tumor cells and normal vasculature (i.e., brain adjacent to tumor) primarily by diffusion from the main tumor mass, rather than directly across brain capillaries. Therefore, prolonged high plasma drug levels will be required to allow for drug diffusion from tumor to brain adjacent to tumor to achieve significant antitumor activity (see Figure 3-3 and 3-4 for example.)

PHARMACOKINETIC CONSIDERATIONS

In addition to understanding the specifics of blood-brain trans-

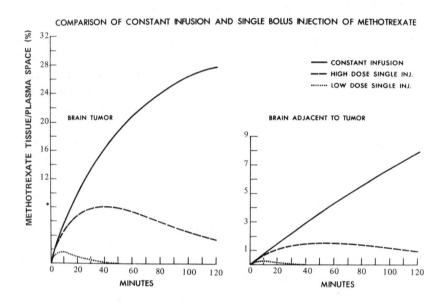

Figure 3-3. Diffusion of Methotrexate into brain tumor and areas of brain adjacent to tumor, indicating uptake into a greatly increased area when drug is administered by constant infusion.

port for chemotherapeutic agents, the physician must be aware of the pharmacokinetics of drugs in the body as a whole. For instance, plasma levels must be maintained for longer periods with polar drugs than with lipid-soluble drugs to achieve significant drug levels in brain adjacent to tumor. After oral, intramuscular (I.M.) or intravenous (I.V.) administration, a drug must first be absorbed and then distributed in body volume. Initial uptake rates, compartmental distribution rates, plasma protein-binding constants, and excretion rates are unique for each drug, and tend to lower the effective plasma level of circulating drug available to an intracerebral tumor.

Protein binding may further reduce the amount of drug

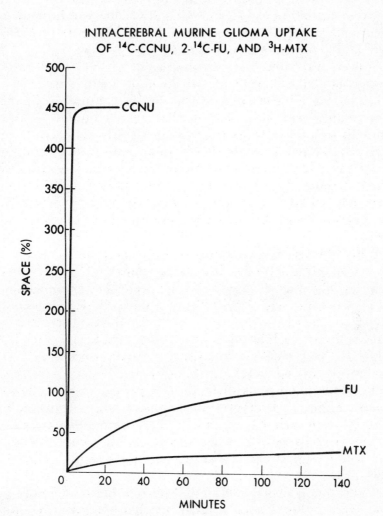

Figure 3-4. Uptake curves for three chemotherapeutic agents into the intracerebral murine glioma.

available to a tumor, either by irreversible binding and removal of drug from the circulation, as occurs with carbamylation and alkylation of the nitrosoureas, or by drug biotransformation while parent drug is reversibly bound (e.g., adsorbed) to plasma protein.[30] Since protein binding of the nitrosoureas increases with increasing lipophilicity, MeCCNU and CCNU would bind to protein and conceivably would break down to inactive products slower and to a greater extent than BCNU.[30]

However, reversible or loose binding of some chemotherapeutic agents to plasma proteins can favorably sustain drug levels in the plasma long enough to increase accumulation in the tumor. Methotrexate is an example of a drug that binds reversibly to protein in a low-affinity reaction; it is easily displaced from protein and quickly establishes a new equilibrium between bound and free drug in plasma.[9] Methotrexate is also recirculated through the enterohepatic system, and since glomerular filtration rather than tubular secretion accounts for its appearance in urine, plasma clearance and excretion of methotrexate are prolonged.

A study of three drugs administered intraperitoneally to mice with intracerebral gliomas illustrates some of the preceding principles. The three drugs were ^{3}H-methotrexate, a nonmetabolized weak organic acid of 454 MW; ^{14}C-fluorouracil (FU), a nonionized pyrimidine analog of 130 MW; and ^{14}C-1-(2-chloroethyl)-3-cyclohexyl-1-nitrosourea (CCNU), a lipid-soluble drug of 234 MW. If these drugs are maintained in plasma at a relatively constant level, the net movement of drug is into the tumor and the pharmacokinetics of such movement are straightforward. Figure 3-4 depicts the uptake and distribution spaces[9, 25, 31, 32] of each drug in intracerebral tumor. Note the progressively increasing distribution spaces and faster equilibration from typical weak organic acid to nonionized to highly lipid-soluble drug.

Methotrexate is distributed in a 14 percent brain-adjacent-to-tumor space in three hours, approaching but not quite reaching equilibrium, while distributing to equilibrium in a space in normal brain of less than 4 percent. It reached an intracellular space of approximately 1 to 2 percent. Saturability of the intracellular

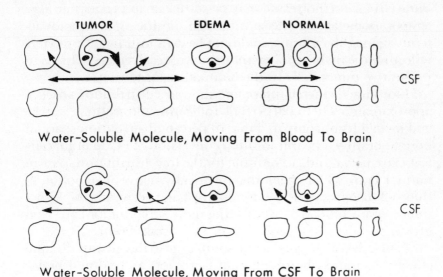

Figure 3-5. Schematic representation of the movement of a water-soluble molecule from blood or CSF into brain and tumor cells. Size of arrows indicates amount of diffusion; "hollow" cells with black dots represent capillaries.

space was not demonstrated although this characteristic of saturability has been demonstrated in L1210 cells.[33] However, cellular binding (probably to dihydrofolate reductase) was quite tight, and at twenty-four hours after a single intraperitoneally (I.P.) injection the tumor/plasma ratio was still formidable, even though the amount of drug remaining in the tumor for twenty-four hours was only 0.5 percent of the injected dose.[9]

Tator, et al. used radioautography following I.P. injection of methotrexate.[34] They found little drug in the extracellular space, which can probably be explained by the rapid initial plasma clearance of methotrexate (t $1/2$ = 7 to 12 min) at the dose used. Their approximation of the percent of drug in tumor was similar to the author's at one hour.[9] Shapiro demonstrated that methotrexate exerts an effect on intracellular incorporation of precursors into DNA in the murine glioma as early as thirty minutes after I.P. injection.[35] This implies that even a small amount of intracellular methotrexate may be sufficient to produce at least temporary metabolic effects, although significant antitumor activity against the glioma could not be demonstrated,[36] probably reflecting the inability of methotrexate to reach effective levels in infiltrative tumor cells in the brain adjacent to tumor.

Fluorouracil entered tumor and showed a distribution space of approximately 110 to 120 percent, indicating intracellular uptake and metabolism, compared to a 10 percent distribution space in normal brain.[31] The intracellular conversion of FU in brain cells was extremely rapid, accounting for the low distribution space in normal brain. The chemotherapeutically active metabolite, 2-fluoro-2'-deoxyuridine-5'-monophosphate, accumulated with a tumor/brain ratio of 17, indicating more rapid tumor entry and greater metabolic conversion than for normal brain.

CCNU, being highly lipid soluble, distributed rapidly and equally in tumor, brain adjacent to tumor, and normal brain, achieving steadystate by seven minutes.[32] The tissue/plasma ratio was 4.3 to 4.9 and CCNU accounted for 15 percent of the ether-soluble fraction. Because of its high lipid solubility, CCNU exchange with brain, brain adjacent to tumor, and tumor was limited by blood flow.

Methotrexate is an example of a polar, water-soluble, weak organic acid that should neither cross the intact blood-brain barrier nor enter nontumor cells appreciably after injection into the CSF. Figure 3-5 schematically depicts how such a molecule would move from blood to brain tumor, normal brain, and CSF (the "sink" effect) and how it could move from CSF to tumor.

Figure 3-6 depicts the manner in which a lipid-soluble agent such as CCNU would move in brain tumor, brain, and CSF. Clearly, CSF instillation of the drug would not achieve significant levels in the tumor because of intracellular and transcapillary exchange as it moved from CSF through brain to tumor. In addition, once the drug arrived at the tumor, loss across tumor capillaries would further reduce tumor drug levels unless there were rapid intracellular binding.

Fluorouracil, being nonionized and metabolized by normal brain and tumor, would have a schematic representation similar

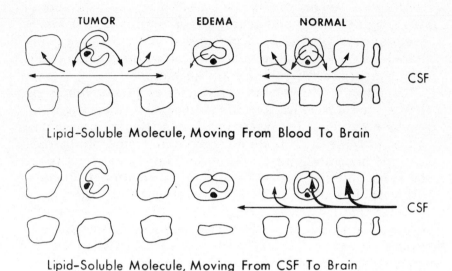

Lipid-Soluble Molecule, Moving From Blood To Brain

Lipid-Soluble Molecule, Moving From CSF To Brain

Figure 3-6. Same as Figure 3-5, except lipid-soluble molecules.

to that of Figure 3-6. It would cross all capillaries but tumor vessels more readily; it would enter and be metabolized by all cells, but tumor cells more rapidly. Although it could diffuse from CSF to brain tumor through the extracellular space, nevertheless much of the drug would enter nontumor cells and cross capillaries on the way, reducing the effective tumor levels and possibly causing neuro- and systemic toxicity.

ROUTES OF ADMINISTRATION

The chemotherapy of brain tumors has not been limited by lack of innovative approaches to drug delivery.[37,38] The failure of previous therapeutic efforts more likely reflects the choice of inactive drugs, inadequate dosage, insufficient frequency of administration, and incomplete knowledge of specific pharmacokinetic factors.

Intra-Arterial

Rationale. Agents can be administered through the carotid artery by single injection, intermittent or continuous infusion, or carotid-jugular perfusion. Intra-arterial (I.A.) administration should achieve a high drug concentration within a tumor that is confined to the carotid territorial distribution.

Theoretically, drugs with rapid rates of plasma-tumor exchange should be efficacious when delivered by the intracarotid arterial route. The ideal drugs for I.A. administration should be lipid-soluble or small nonionized molecules, since they would have the maximum entry into surrounding tissue per passage through capillaries in tumor and brain. In addition, with cross-compression of a contralateral vertebral or carotid artery, even greater tissue entry could be obtained. This approach would permit administration of lower doses and hence lessen systemic toxicity.

Limitations. Intra-arterial administration has two major limitations, neurotoxicity, i.e., direct damage to brain within the infused area, and anatomical limitations of the field of infusion. Quite apart from the pH and osmolarity of the infusate, a drug may be directly neurotoxic, although this complication should be avoidable by suitable preclinical toxicity studies in animals.

Of greater importance is the limitation imposed by the distribution of the infusate within the target area. Rush, et al.[39] studied the anatomic and distributional factors related to I.A. infusion, using a cadaver flow model and the distribution of Evans blue dye in patients. Dye injected at 1 cc per minute through a 23 gauge needle remained in a long thread without mixing over a distance of 5 or more cm. Injection into the midstream missed proximal branches, and with injection adjacent to the vessel wall, most or all of the contrast medium entered the first branch encountered. They concluded that the only practical method of achieving good mixing was introduction of the agent in a jet stream, i.e., rapid injection through a small orifice. Newton[40] studied the distribution of fluorescein within a tumor and reported an uneven and irregular distribution following I.A. injection.

Another serious limitation of I.A. infusion is the bilaterality of a substantial number of gliomas and their frequent location within areas supplied by two or more major cerebral arteries, e.g., middle cerebral artery and posterior cerebral artery.

Technique. Correct localization is imperative in all I.A. techniques. In the vertebral artery, correct placement is determined either by open operation or by injection of radio-opaque medium. In the carotid system, localization becomes critical. Whether the technique is percutaneous cannulation or open arteriotomy, insurance of flow into the internal carotid artery must be verified by injection of either an opaque medium (which might irritate brain and tumor capillaries) or a substance that can be visualized in the ophthalmic artery distribution. The author has used fluorescein,[41] but dyes that can be visualized under ambient light are equally satisfactory.[42]

A drug can be administered intermittently or by continuous infusion. Percutaneous placement of a needle or catheter is suitable for administration over a period of several minutes to an hour. For longer administration, i.e. infusion, placement of a catheter is essential to prevent damage to the intima by the inflexible needle and to prevent displacement of the needle from the artery. The Seldinger technique of catheterization is suitable for cervical placement of an internal carotid catheter,[43] and the author has used a large bore needle without the more refined Seldinger technique.[41] Transfemoral catheterization of the internal carotid artery has not been used for long-term infusion, perhaps because of the increased danger of infection in the genital-rectal area and the risk of deep venous thrombosis in the catheterized extremity. Many authors advocate the direct placement of a catheter, introducing it through either the common carotid artery or the superior thyroid artery. Nelsen, et al. give an excellent description of catheter fixation.[44]

Injection by hand is suitable for short-term injections. For injections over a period of time and for long-term infusions, several techniques are available. Espinar, et al.[45] used simple gravity. The authors have used the Barron pump,[41] originally described by Tucker and Talley.[46] An excellent and easily managed infusion apparatus is the Fenwal bag,[41] which employs an inflated cuff surrounding a plastic bag containing the infusate. This method is easily managed by nursing personnel, and when the bag is properly filled, avoids the potential complication of air embolism. Syringe pumps have shown remarkable versatility and were used extensively by Mahaley and Woodhall.[47] Sullivan introduced a miniaturized clock-driven infusion apparatus that hangs around the patient's neck in a special vest designed for ambulatory patients on both inpatient and outpatient basis.[48,49] Bags containing the infusate are mailed to the patient, and with rather simple directions either he or his family can change the bag; the patient can remain independent of professional care for extended periods.

Certain agents, because of decomposition, cannot be mixed and administered over long periods of time. Unfortunately, many of the effective cell-cycle-nonspecific agents currently in use are not stable in solution for extended periods, but this problem can be circumvented if efficacy of I.A. therapy can be demonstrated.

Perfusion. Woodhall and Mahaley, with their collaborators at Duke, were pioneers in the isolated perfusion technique for the chemotherapy of brain tumors.[50,52] Discouraged by their results, they later switched to arterial infusion. Unfortunately, the isolation-perfusion technique using one or both internal carotid arteries and jugular veins does not approach a closed system because of spillover of the infusate to pericranial tissues and the return of venous blood to the systemic circulation by way of the perivertebral venous plexus. Further, isolation of both carotid arteries involves risks and poses technical difficulties.[53]. Feind, et al.,[54] using bilateral common carotid and internal jugular vein cannulation, improved vascular isolation of the head and neck by applying a tourniquet to the base of the neck while occluding the internal vertebral venous plexus with an epidural balloon. Because of the technical difficulties attending this procedure, it has not been pursued. Moss[55] accomplished total perfusion of the brain in the calf by perfusing one common carotid artery at a pressure of 20 mm of Hg greater than systemic pressure, and angiograms demonstrated reverse flow in the distribution of the contralateral carotid artery and both vertebral arteries. This method has not been applied to man. There seems to be little advantage in using I.A. perfusion instead of infusion when risks are weighed against potential benefits.

Complications. The I.A. administration of chemotherapeutic agents has been attended by many complications, the great majority being associated with long-term infusions through indwelling catheters. Neurological deficits, both transient and permanent, can be attributed in some cases to arterial spasm either from the drug or from the effect of the indwelling catheter.[56] With all long-term infusions, an additional problem has been infection at the cutaneous exit of the catheter, whether in the cervical or thoracic regions.

The major complication of arterial catheterization has been thrombosis of the internal carotid artery. In the majority of instances, carotid thrombosis has been an unexpected finding by angiography or at postmortem examination.[41] The incidence is no doubt related to the type of catheter and the duration of its presence in the artery. Benson, et al.[57] have advised the use of catheters of the smallest possible size, since a small catheter becomes excluded from the blood stream by a circumferential sheath of fibrin thrombus which fixes it to the vessel wall. Occlusion of the catheter tip by blood products is avoidable by a mechanism providing constant efflux from the catheter tip and by the addition of heparin to the infusate. Meticulous attention to detail can significantly reduce the occurrence of air embolism and thrombosis.

Another common and potentially serious complication is displacement of the catheter. Although no instances have been reported, the catheter tip can be advanced too far into the intracranial carotid artery, increasing the risk of thrombosis and even perforation of the vessel wall. Of more practical importance is displacement of the catheter tip from the vessel lumen with consequent bleeding and leakage of the infusate into the perivascular soft tissues. Both may produce swelling and the risk of venous and airway obstruction.

Increased intracranial pressure subsequent to treatment is not unique to I.A. therapy, but possibly the drug concentrations achieved by I.A. administration pose a particular problem in this regard.[58,59] Increased intracranial pressure can occur as a consequence of tumor necrosis, with or without additional cerebral edema caused by neurotoxicity of the infused agent. The current availability of means to combat cerebral edema lessens this threat.

Transitory and permanent ophthalmoplegia have occurred in patients receiving intracarotid infusions of nitrogen mustard and the vinca alkaloids.[41,60]

Vasculitis in dogs given a high I.A. dose of BCNU has been reported recently, which may dampen enthusiasm for intracarotid therapy with BCNU in man.[61]

Agents administered by I.A. methods. A number of agents have been administered by various I.A. techniques, none with outstanding success. Among the agents used have been methotrexate,[59] vinblastine sulfate,[41,62] vincristine sulfate,[60,63,64] nitrogen mustard[53,58] phenylalanine mustard,[65] triethylenethiophosphoramide (Thiotepa®)[66,67] and 5-bromo-2'-deoxyuridine (BUdR).[68] BUdR has been used only in conjunction with radiation therapy, whereas several of the agents listed above have been used both singly and with radiation therapy.

Intraventricular and Intrathecal

Rationale. Since the ependyma and arachnoid appear to present little restriction to the movement of molecules between CSF and brain extracellular space,[7,9] direct intrathecal (I.T.) and intraventricular administration of chemotherapeutic agents have been advocated for molecules too large to pass the blood-brain barrier, as well as for drugs producing excessive systemic toxicity or drugs that are rapidly inactivated in blood. The obvious advantage of achieving and in maintaining a high level of drug in the CSF is, in most cases, lessened by the tumor's location deep within the brain, at a distance 2 to 4 cm from the CSF. Since, theoretically, a drug introduced into the CSF should possess a diffusion coefficient favoring rapid transit through the tortuous extracellular space of intact brain, one could arbitrarily eliminate such drugs as L-asparaginase because of molecular size. Drugs with smaller molecules, such as the pyrimidine and purine analogs, would be more reasonable. Even the use of methotrexate would seem to be contraindicated in many situations because of its molecular size (454 MW) and ionization.

Limitations. Intrathecally administered polar molecules move by bulk flow from the lumbar subarachnoid space to the basal cisterns and then to the cerebral convexities. Absorption then occurs through the arachnoid villi into the venous blood of the sagittal sinus. This pattern can be modified unpredictably by intracranial tumors, and proper distribution requires special techniques to insure movement of the drug to its site of action. Clearly, the location of a tumor near the ventricular rather than the subarachnoid surface would severely compromise the effectiveness of I.T. administered chemotherapeutic agents.

Simple lumbar injection of methotrexate has been highly successful in the treatment of meningeal leukemia. However, (1) meningeal leukemia is almost invariably accompanied by communicating hydrocephalus with its abnormal flow pattern and reflux into the cerebral ventricles; and (2) access of the drug to cells that are either free floating or enmeshed in leptomeninges presents a problem entirely different from drug delivery to a solid tumor. Although methotrexate controls the manifestations of meningeal leukemia and at the same time eliminates leukemic cells as determined by CSF cystology, recurrences (unexplainable by hematogenous metastasis) indicate survival of at least a few leukemic cells. These may occur either because the drug failed to reach all leukemic cells at effective concentrations or because treatment is stopped before elimination of the last cell.

The author conducted a Phase II study of continuous (thirty-six hour) high dose methotrexate infusion using either the spinal subarachnoid space or a ventricular reservoir, followed by systemic leucovorin (citrovorum factor) rescue (see Chapter Seven), but he has since used this approach sparingly because of the kinetic characteristics of gliomas and the pharmacokinetics and pharmacodynamics of methotrexate.

Intrathecal therapy offers little advantage unless the tumor is in the path of subarachnoid CSF, because normal CSF dynamics are such that I.T. administered drugs do not enter the ventricular system to a significant extent.[11] Intraventricular therapy, with a reservoir, or by ventricular-lumbar perfusion, has the obvious

advantage over I.T. administration of delivering high drug levels
in close proximity to the brain. However, the effectiveness of the
drug entering from CSF into brain and tumor will be dependent
on (1) the diffusion coefficient of the drug, (2) capillary permeability, (3) drug stability in CSF, (4) the location of the tumor
relative to the ventricular surface, and (5) the drug's neurotoxicity.

As mentioned previously, in addition to arachnoid villus absorption, capillary permeability in tumor and in normal brain
can account for significant systemic absorption of drug from
brain and tumor ECS with resultant systemic toxicity. For a drug
with the molecular size of fluorouracil, at least 13 percent of
intraventricular drug could leak across normal capillaries, and
possibly 10 percent across tumor capillaries.[26]

One goal of ventricular perfusion is to achieve significant tumoricidal drug levels in the brain adjacent to tumor where the
infiltrative "fingers" of a tumor exist without highly permeable
vessels. To do this with a drug such as methotrexate, with the
tumor at a depth of 2 cm from the ventricle, a piece of brain 4 cm
in ventricular-subarachnoid breadth would have to be perfused
on both the ventricular and subarachnoid surfaces for forty-eight
hours to achieve 8 percent of CSF concentration at a depth of 2 cm.
Figure 3-7 depicts the diffusion of methotrexate into such a piece
of tissue. If ventricular-lumbar perfusion was carried out and
little drug was available to the cortical subarachnoid space (such
as in cases of hydrocephalus, hemispheral edema, and meningitis), then perfusions would have to continue for eight to ten
days in order to achieve similar concentrations at a distance of 3 to
5 cm from the ventricle. Unfortunately, perfusions of this duration may result in neurotoxicity.

Neurotoxicity constitutes a significant factor in selecting drugs
for I.T. administration. For instance, vinblastine sulfate, while
well tolerated following vascular injection, is markedly neurotoxic following intracisternal administration in the dog.[69] Other
drugs, e.g., methotrexate, are relatively nonneurotoxic by comparison even when administered in massive doses,[70] although
reports of idiosyncratic neurotoxicity have appeared.[71] Walker, et
al.[72] have attempted to relate the toxicity of I.T. drugs to their

THEORETICAL DIFFUSIONAL DRUG DISTRIBUTION IN BRAIN FOR METHOTREXATE AFTER 48 hrs OF VENTRICULAR PERFUSION

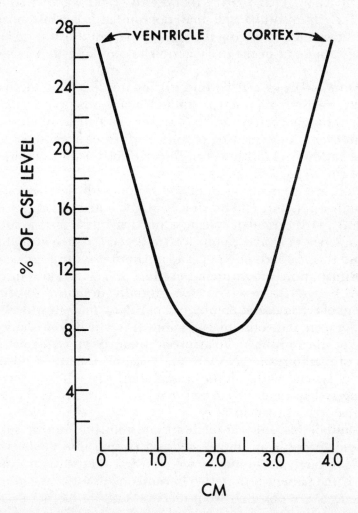

Figure 3-7. Curve showing the theoretical concentrations of Methotrexate in brain tissue at varying distances from the ventricle after forty eight hours of ventricular perfusion.

ionic content. In dogs, the only drug causing convulsions was methotrexate, and although this is rare in clinical experience, it has occurred in the author's hands. For this reason concurrent administration of prophylactic anticonvulsants is advisable.

Drugs that do not cross the blood-brain barrier will be removed by bulk flow. In addition, weak organic drugs such as methotrexate can be actively removed by the choroid plexus as demonstrated by Rubin, et al.[73] Drugs that readily cross the blood-brain barrier (i.e., lipid-soluble and small nonionized drugs) lose much of their advantage following intraventricular administration because of rapid exit of the drug across the capillaries in normal brain.

Technique. Drugs can be injected intermittently by lumbar puncture, by cisternal puncture, through a previously placed burr hole, or through a reservoir. All of these routes are available for infusion over a longer period of time. Perfusion, using separate sites for inflow and outflow, can be performed using combinations of sites related to the target area.

Newton, et al.,[74] treating childhood tumors with methotrexate, used lumbar puncture and previously placed burr holes for injection into the ventricular system. Ommaya[75] described a subcutaneous reservoir and pump for sterile access to ventricular CSF, and this has become a popular apparatus for intraventricular administration, intermittent injection, and continuous infusion. Although the reservoir was initially designed for the treatment of cryptococcal meningitis, oncolytic agents are ideally suited for percutaneous injection into this mushroom-shaped capsule of silicon rubber. To assure adequate mixing and distribution of methotrexate, Norrell and Wilson[76] used the Pudenz shunting system with unidirectional flow. A unidirectional shunting system creates a current that can be directed to the desired area over a broad surface.

The author has infused methotrexate into the lumbar subarachnoid space via an indwelling catheter and into the lateral ventricle through an Ommaya reservoir using a Harvard infusion pump. If the patient is protected by anticonvulsant medication, no ill effects are observed from massive doses of methotrexate followed in twenty-four to thirty-six hours by systemic leucovorin rescue. In this and other systems, one can obtain an approximation of the bulk flow of the administered molecules by observing the distribution of concomitantly injected or infused RISA using serial scintiscans.

Perfusion. Cerebrospinal perfusion provides a novel approach for the delivery of substances normally excluded by the blood-brain barrier. The method's complexity detracts from its general applicability, but in certain special situations it may provide an effective method of adjuvant chemotherapy.

Ommaya, et al.[77] first reported the perfusion of oncolytic agents using techniques long practiced by physiologists. Depending upon the tumor's site, they established a perfusion system from ventricle to lumbar subarachnoid space, from lateral ventricle to lateral ventricle, from temporal horn to the body of the lateral ventricle, and from the tumor cavity to the lateral ventricle.

Subsequently, Rubin, et al.[78,79] reported further experience with CSF perfusions. A cannula was placed either in the frontal horn or in the tumor bed (in cases where a fistula had been created between the tumor bed and the adjacent ventricle) and a second cannula was placed elsewhere in the CSF space to provide an outflow route. They reported their experience using methotrexate and 8-azaguanine perfused through combinations of Ommaya reservoirs and spinal cannulas. In the case of lipid-insoluble and highly ionized substances, e.g. methotrexate, egress of the molecule from CSF occurs largely by bulk flow, and the rate of bulk flow is determined by the effective hypostatic pressure, i.e., the difference between intraventricular and superior sagittal sinus venous pressures. They minimized systemic leakage of drug by perfusing with the outflow cannula set at the right heart level (0 cm H 0). Using inulin as an indicator of bulk flow, they determined that absorption was directly related to the surface area exposed in the circuit and to the volume of the perfusate. They suggested that drugs possessing small therapeutic indices could be used to advantage by carefully selecting the route and frequency of administration.

Perfusion provides one means of exploiting relative pharmacological barriers to retain rather than exclude active compounds. The penetration of a drug such as methotrexate occurs by diffusion independently of intraventricular pressure. At higher flow rates the inflow concentration approaches the effective drug concentration, and it has not proved necessary to increase the inflow rate beyond 3 ml/minute.

Complications. With long-term infusions and perfusions, the danger of infection is evident. Demyelination and seizures have occurred.[71] The chemical nature of the drug as well as the effect of the diluent may be responsible for side-effects with individual agents, such as meningeal irritation, and paraplegia occurring with methotrexate.[80,81]

A potential complication, as yet unreported, is injury to neural tissue secondary to CSF manipulation. Bunge and Settlage[82] produced lasting neurological deficits and histological lesions in cats by forcibly injecting CSF into the cisterna magna. More recently, forceful injection of CSF withdrawn from the lumbar subarachnoid space has been reported as a means of relieving pain.[45] In light of these reports, I.T. injection should be made slowly.

Intratumor

Rationale. Effective local (topical) chemotherapy presumes that an agent will move freely throughout the tumor from its point of application and at the same time produce no adverse effects on uninvolved intradural structures. If experience with topical chemotherapy of extracranial tumors serves as any guide, this method has little potential for intracranial tumors.

Limitations. Theoretically, a water-soluble drug, unless it binds tightly to brain tumor cell membranes or enters cells, would leak across tumor capillaries into the systemic circulation lowering its concentration within the tumor. This might be of little practical importance if the dose were sufficiently high to exert an antitumor effect, but a lipid-soluble drug would move especially rapidly from intratumor sites to the systemic circulation.

Technique. Selverstone[84] describes a stereotaxic technique for the local injection of 8-azaguanine. Ringkjob[85] treated gliomas and metastatic carcinomas by the local application of Thiotepa and 5-FU. He described several techniques using both liquid and powdered agents administered through a catheter left in the tumor cavity at the time of operation. He observed no harmful effects, and no histological changes were apparent in normal brain at the time of postmortem examination.

Raskind and Weiss injected methotrexate into tumor cavities through an Ommaya reservoir placed at the time of surgery.[86] Although the heterogeneity of their patient population precluded an evaluation of the drug's effectiveness, one of the authors of this book (C.B.W.) examined his postmortem specimens and was impressed with the striking necrosis present in the shell of tumor surrounding the surgically created cavity. Garfield and Dayan have given up to 1250 mg of methotrexate daily for four to ten days by postoperative intracavitary catheter and reported modest chemotherapeutic responses in nine patients.[87]

Methotrexate may be an ideal drug in this respect since it moves well through the extracellular space of both tumor and surrounding brain, and one can achieve extremely high concentrations locally within the limits of systemic toxicity. Its disadvantage as a primary mode of therapy lies in its cell-cycle specificity in tumors of low growth fraction. As an immediate adjunct to surgical removal, the local application of oncolytic drugs probably deserves some further study.

DRUG ACTION

The last consideration in planning effective brain tumor chemotherapy — drug action — might more properly have been the first. To be maximally effective, various classes of drugs must be delivered differently and a basic knowledge of brain and tumor pharmacokinetics must precede any choice of chemotherapeutic agent and route of administration.

As outlined in the discussion of Bruce's work in Chapter One, fundamentally there are two classes of tumoricidal drugs, cell-cycle-specific (CCS; including phase-specific) and cell-cycle-non-specific (CCNS).[88] The former interfere with the progression of cells through the cell cycle, usually by inhibiting DNA synthesis, and the latter with the functional integrity of DNA in noncycling as well as in cycling cells. The CCS agents interfere with movement of the cell through one or more phases of the cell cycle, usually S phase or M phase; the majority are purine and pyrimidine analogs, antimetabolites, or vinca alkaloids. The CCNS agents interfere directly with DNA; these include the alkylating and intercalating agents.

To be most effective, CCS drugs must be given repeatedly or continuously over a prolonged period to effect repeated cell-kill of cycling cells.[89] During each exposure to an effective drug, a percentage of the dividing cell population is killed. In theory, all dividing cells could be destroyed eventually by repeated drug administration in the absence of systemic toxicity, enzyme adaptation, or cell mutation and resistance. In practice, the emergence of a drug-resistant population often leads to tumor regrowth. In addition, only a small percentage (30%) of cells may actually be in cycle during even prolonged therapeutic periods. Thus not even a one log cell-kill might be expected from even the most aggressive therapy with CCS agents.

Pharmacokinetically, CCS drugs should enter and distribute rapidly in tumor and in brain adjacent to tumor; ideally, these agents should cross the normal blood-brain barrier in order to reach infiltrating tumor cells some distance from the main tumor mass. Since drugs must be given repeatedly, the route of delivery should be suitable for long-term administration.

The CCNS drugs attack noncycling as well as cycling cells by their effects on nucleic acids through alkylation, binding, or intercalation. Since much of the damage they cause is reversible with time, or is negated by DNA repair mechanisms, ideally they should be suitable for repeated administration over prolonged periods. Fortunately, many CCNS agents are lipid soluble. For these drugs, either a high dose I.V. injection over thirty to sixty minutes or brief intracarotid arterial infusion for five to twenty minutes would be expected to attain high tumor and brain-adjacent-to-tumor levels with tolerable toxicity.[30] Unless a lipid soluble drug binds very rapidly within tumor cells, no advantage would be gained by intracarotid administration (as opposed to I.V. injection) because exchange across the capillaries of the brain, when coupled with a rapidly falling plasma drug level, will be so rapid that the drug will cross back into the blood from the tumor as it seeks to equilibrate with the now lower plasma drug level. These factors must be evaluated to ascertain the optimal route of administration for each agent to be so used.

Combination therapy with chemotherapeutic agents, to be effective, should follow the rules cited above for single agents. Theoretically, this approach deserves serious consideration in brain tumors, particularly in view of recent successes in leukemia, lymphoma, and lung cancer. Drug combinations offer distinct chemotherapeutic advantages if the drugs have different toxic effects, different modes of action, and if their combined use delays the emergence of drug-resistant tumor cells. Because human brain tumors contain a high proportion of noncycling cells, effective combinations of drugs should include one or more effective CCNS agents. Obviously, combination chemotherapy should, in general, incorporate CCNS agents known to be effective in single agent Phase II trials. However, CCS agents, which may only achieve a one log cell, kill, need not demonstrate significant experimental animal or human increased survival as single agents to be effective in drug combination therapy.

REFERENCES

1. Brightman, M.W., Klatzo, I., Olssen, Y., and Reese, T.S.: The blood-brain barrier to proteins under normal and pathological conditions. *J Neurol Sci, 10*:215, 1970.
2. Fenstermacher, J.D., and Johnson, J.A.: Filtration and reflection coefficients of the rabbit blood-brain barrier. *Am J Physiol, 211*:341, 1966.
3. Crone, C.: The permeability of brain capillaries to nonelectrolytes. *Acta Physiol Scand, 64*:407, 1965.
4. Fenstermacher, J.D., Rall, D.P., Patlak, C.S., and Levin, V.: Ventriculocisternal perfusion as a technique for analysis of brain capillary permeability and extracellular transport. In Crone, C. and Lassen, N.A. (Eds.): *Capillary Permeability*. Proceedings of the Alfred Benzon Symposium II, 1969. Copenhagen, Munksgaard, 1970, pp. 483-490.
5. Levin, V.A. and Patlak, C.S.: A compartmental analysis of ^{24}Na kinetics in rat cerebrum, sciatic nerve, and cerebrospinal fluid. *J Physiol (Lond), 224*:559, 1972.

6. Levin, V.A., Fenstermacher, J.D., and Patlak, C.: Sucrose and inulin space measurements of cerebral cortex in four mammalian species. *Am J Physiol, 219*:1528, 1970.

7. Brodie, B.B., Kurz, H., and Schanker, L.S.: The importance of dissociation constant and lipid-solubility in influencing the passage of drugs into the cerebrospinal fluid. *J Pharmacol Exp Ther, 130*:20, 1960.

8. Rall, D.P., and Zubrod, C.S.: Mechanisms of drug absorption and excretion: passage of drugs in and out of the central nervous system. *Annu Rev Pharmacol, 2*:109, 1962.

9. Levin, V.A., Clancy, T.P., Ausman, J.I., and Rall, D.P.: Uptake and distribution of ³H-methotrexate by the murine ependymoblastoma. *J Natl Cancer Inst, 48*:875, 1972.

10. Davson, H., Kleeman, C.R., and Levin, E.: Blood-brain barrier and extracellula space. *J Physiol (Lond), 159*:67, 1961.

11. DiChiro, G.: Movement of the cerebrospinal fluid in human beings. *Nature (Lond), 204*:290, 1964.

12. Rieselbach, R.E., DiChiro, G., Freireich, E.J., and Rall, D.P.: Subarachnoid distribution of drugs after lumbar injection. *N Engl J Med, 267*:1273, 1962.

13. Hoshino, T., Barker, M., Wilson, C.B., et al.: Cell kinetics of human gliomas. *J Neurosurg, 37*:15, 1972.

14. Ausman, J.I. and Levin, V.A.: Intra- and extravascular distribution of standard drug molecules in brain tumor and brain. In Drake, C.G., and Duvoisin, R. (Eds.): *Fourth International Congress of Neurological Surgery,* 1969; International Congress Series, no. 193. New York, Excerpta Medica Foundation, 1970, p. 41.

15. Hadjidimos, A., Steingass, U., Fischer, F., et al.: The effects of dexamethasone on rCBF and cerebral vasomotor response in brain tumors. *Eur Neurol, 10*:25, 1973.

16. Sivachenko, T.P., Zozulia, Iu.A., and Spiridonova, M.V.: Determination of regional cerebral circulation in cases of cerebral tumors by means of Xe-133. *Med Radiol (Mosk), 17*:36, 1972.

17. Levin, V.A., Dove, M.A., Landahl H.: The permeability characteristics of the brain adjacent to intracerebral rodent tumors. *Arch Neurol 32*:785-791, 1975.

18. Bakay, L.: Basic aspects of brain tumor localization by radioactive substances. *J Neurosurg, 27*:239, 1967.

19. Cohn, H.J., and Soiderer, M.N.: Tissue vascularity in positive and negative brain scans. *J Nucl Med, 10*:553, 1969.

20. Hirano, A., Becker, N., and Zimmerman, H.: Pathological alterations in the cerebral endothelial cell barrier to peroxidase. *Arch Neurol, 20*:300, 1969.

21. Long, D.: Capillary ultrastructure and the blood-brain barrier in human brain tumors. In *Sixty International Congress of Neuropathology.* Paris, Masson et Cie, 1970, pp. 994-996.

22. Nystrom, S.: Pathological changes in blood vessels of human glioblastoma

multiforme. Comparative studies using plastic casting, angiography, light microscopy and electron microscopy, and with reference to some other brain tumors. *Acta Pathol Microbiol Scand, 49*: Suppl. 137, 1960.

23. Shuttleworth, E.C., Jr.: Barrier phenomena in brain tumors. In Bingham, W.G., Jr. (Ed.): *Recent Advances in Brain Tumor Research (Progress in Experimental Tumor Research, Vol. 17)* Basel, Karger, 1972, pp.279-290.

24. Torack, R.M.: Ultrastructure of capillary reaction to brain tumors. *Arch Neurol, 5*:416, 1961.

25. Levin, V.A., Ausman, J., and Chadwick, M.: Pharmacokinetics of standard molecules and chemotherapeutic agents in a murine glioma. *Proc Am Assoc Cancer Res, 13*:95, 1972.

26. Levin, V.A.: Unpublished observations, 1969-1973.

27. Ausman, J.I., Levin, V.A., and Brown, W.: Unpublished observations, 1969.

28. Kabra, P.M., Levin, V.A., and Freeman, M.A.: Unpublished observations.

29. Oliverio, V.T., Vietzke, W.M., Williams, M.K., and Adamson, R.H.: The absorption, distribution, excretion, and biotransformation of the carcinostatic 1-(2-chloroethyl)-3-cyclohexyl-1-nitrosourea in animals. *Cancer Res, 30*:1330, 1970.

30. Levin, V.A., Kabra, P.M.: Brain and brain tumor pharmacokinetics of BCNU and CCNU following i. v. and intracarotid artery (i.c.a.) administration. Proc. Am. Assoc. *Cancer Res., 16*:19, 1975.

31. Levin, V.A., and Chadwick, M.: Distribution of 5-fluorouracil-2-^{14}C and its metabolites in a murine glioma. *J Natl Cancer Inst 49*:1577, 1972.

32. Levin, V.A., Shapiro, W.R., Clancy, T.P., and Oliverio, V.T.: The uptake, distribution, and antitumor activity of 1-(2-chloroethyl)-3-cyclohexyl-1-nitrosourea in the murine glioma. *Cancer Res, 30*:2451, 1970.

33. Goldman, I.D., Lichtenstein, N.S., and Oliverio, V.T.: Carrier-mediated transport of the folic acid analogue, methotrexate, in the L1210 leukemia cell. *J Biol Chem, 243*:500, 1968.

34. Tator, C.H.: Chemotherapy of brain tumors. Uptake of tritiated methotrexate by a transplantable intracerebral ependymoblastoma in mice. *J Neurosurg, 37*:1, 1972.

35. Shapiro, W.R.: The effect of chemotherapeutic agents on incorporation of DNA precursors by experimental brain tumors. *Cancer Res., 32*:2178, 1972.

36. Shapiro, W.R., Ausman, J.I., and Rall, D.P.: Studies on the chemotherapy of experimental brain tumors: evaluation of 1,3-bis-(2-chloroethyl)-1-nitrosourea, cyclophosphamide, mithramycin, and methotrexate. *Cancer Res, 30*:2401, 1970.

37. Broder, L.E., and Rall, D.P.: Chemotherapy of brain tumors. In Bingham, W.G., Jr. (Ed.): *Recent Advances in Brain Tumor Research (Progress in Experimental Tumor Research, Vol. 17)*, Basel, Karger, 1972, pp. 373-399.

38. Shapiro, W.R., and Ausman, J.I.: The chemotherapy of brain tumors: a clinical and experimental review. In Plum, F. (Ed.); *Recent Advances in Neurology*, Philadelphia, Davis, 1969, pp. 150-235.

39. Rush, B.F., Jr., Horie, N., and Klein, N.W.: Intra-arterial infusion of the

head and neck. Anatomic and distributional problems. *Am J Surg, 110*:510, 1965.

40. Newton, K.A.: The distribution of dyes and fluorescent substances by the blood stream within tumors. *Br J Radiol, 38*:224, 1965.

41. Wilson, C.B.: Chemotherapy of brain tumors by continuous arterial infusion. *Surgery, 55*:640, 1964.

42. Engeset, A., Brennhovd, I., and Stovner, J.: Intra-arterial infusions in cancer chemotherapy. A technique for testing drug distribution. *Lancet, 1*:1382, 1962.

43. Dean, M.R.E., Newton, K.A., and Swann, G.F.: Percutaneous intraarterial chemotherapy in the treatment of intracranial neoplasms: a review of 36 cases. *Br J Radiol, 40*:828, 1967.

44. Nelsen, T.S., Eigenbrodt, E.H., and Bagshaw, M.A.: Low-flow fail-safe intra-arterial infusion. *Arch Surg, 87*:640, 1963.

45. Espiner, H.J., Vowles, K.D.J., and Walker, R.M.: Cancer chemotherapy by intra-arterial infusion. A preliminary report concerning tumors of the head and neck. *Lancet, 1*:177, 1962.

46. Tucker, J.L., Jr. and Talley, R.W.: Prolonged intra-arterial chemotherapy for inoperable cancer: a technique. *Cancer, 14*:493, 1961.

47. Mahaley, M.S., Jr., and Woodhall, B.: Regional chemotherapeutic perfusion and infusion of brain and face tumors. *Ann Surg, 166*:266, 1967.

48. Watkins, E.: Chronometric infusor — an apparatus for protracted ambulatory infusion therapy. *N Engl J Med, 269*:850, 1963.

49. Watkins, E., Jr., and Sullivan, R.D.: Cancer chemotherapy by prolonged arterial infusion. *Surg Gynecol Obstet, 118*:3, 1964.

50. Mahaley, M.S., Jr., and Woodhall, B.: An evaluation of plasma levels of alkylating agents during regional chemotherapeutic perfusions. *J Surg Res, 1*:285, 1961.

51. Woodhall, B., and Mahaley, M.S., Jr.: Isolated perfusion in treatment of advanced carcinoma. *Am J Surg, 105*:624, 1963.

52. Woodhall, B., Hall, K., Mahaley, S., Jr., and Jackson, J.: Chemotherapy of brain cancer: experimental and clinical studies in localized hypothermic cerebral perfusion. *Ann Surg, 150*:640, 1959.

53. Perese, D.M., Day, C.E., and Chardack, W.M.: Chemotherapy of brain tumors by intra-arterial infusion. *J Neurosurg, 19*:215, 1962.

54. Feind, C.R., Herter, F., and Markowitz, A.: Improvements in isolation head perfusion. *Am J Surg, 106*:777, 1963.

55. Moss, G.: Total perfusion of brain with cancer chemotherapeutic agents. *Neurology (Minneap), 15*:531, 1965.

56. Swann, G.F.: Recent advances in neuroradiology. *Postgrad Med J, 37*:385, 1961.

57. Benson, J.W., Kiehn, C.L., and Holden, W.D.: Cancer chemotherapy by arterial infusion. *Arch Surg, 87*:125, 1963.

58. French, J.D., West, P.M., Von Amerongen, F.K., and Magoun, H.W.: Effects of intracarotid administration of nitrogen mustard on normal brain and

brain tumors. *J Neurosurg, 9*:378, 1952.
59. Greenhouse, A.H., Neuberger, K.T., and Bowerman, D.L.: Brain damage after intracarotid infusion of methotrexate. *Arch Nuerol, 11*:618, 1964.
60. Owens, G., Javid, R., Tallon, M., et al.: Arterial infusion chemotherapy of primary gliomas. A report of thirty cases. *JAMA, 186*:802, 1963.
61. DeWys, W.D., and Fowler, E.H.: Report of vasculitis and blindness after intracarotid injection of 1,3-bis(2-chloroethyl)-1-nitrosourea (BCNU;NSC-409962) in dogs. *Cancer Chemother Rep, 57*:33, 1973.
62. Mealey, J., Jr.: Treatment of malignant cerebral astrocytomas by intra-arterial infusion of vinblastine. *Cancer Chemother Rep, 20*:121, 1962.
63. Owens, G., Javid, R., and Belmusto, L.: Chemotherapy of glioblastoma multiforme. In deVet, A.C. (Ed.): *Proceedings of the Third International Congress Neurol Surg*, 1965, International Congress Series, no. 110. New York, Excerpta Medica Foundation, 1966, pp. 752-755.
64. Owens, G., Javid, R., Belmusto, L., et al.: Intra-arterial vincristine therapy of primary gliomas. *Cancer, 18*:756, 1965.
65. Ariel, I.M.: Intra-arterial chemotherapy for metastatic cancer to the brain. *Am J Surg, 102*:647, 1961.
66. Davis, P.L., and Shumway, M.H.: Thio-TEPA in treatment of metastatic cerebral malignancy. *JAMA, 175*:714, 1961.
67. Mark, V.H., Kjellberg, R.N., Ojemann, R.G., and Soloway, A.H.: Treatment of malignant brain tumors with alkylating agents. *Neurology (Minneap), 10*:772, 1960.
68. Sano, K., Hoshino, T., Nagai, M., et al.: Studies on a radiosensitizer (5-bromo-2'-deoxyuridine) in the treatment of malignant brain tumors. *Neurol Med Chir (Tokyo), 8*:227, 1966.
69. Hockey, A.A., and Mealey, J., Jr.: Effects of intracisternal vinblastine in dogs. *Surg Forum, 16*:427, 1965.
70. Lampkin, B.C., Higgins, G.R., and Hammond, D.: Absence of neurotoxicity following massive intrathecal administration of methotrexate. *Cancer, 20*:1780, 1967.
71. Shapiro, W.R., Chernik, N.L., and Posner, J.B.: Necrotizing encephalopathy following intraventricular instillation of methotrexate. *Arch Neruol, 28*:96, 1973.
72. Walker, M.D., Dalgard, D.W., and Hurwitz, B.S.: The toxicity of intrathecal drugs and their ionic content. *Proc Amer Assoc Cancer Res, 10*:97, 1969.
73. Rubin, R., Owens, E., and Rall, D.: Transport of methotrexate by the choroid plexus. *Cancer Res, 28*:689, 1968.
74. Newton, W.A., Jr., Sayers, M.P., and Samuels, L.D.: Intrathecal methotrexate (NSC-740) therapy for brain tumors in children. *Cancer Chemother Rep, 52*:257, 1968.
75. Ommaya, A.K.: Subcutaneous reservoir and pump for sterile access to ventricular cerebrospinal fluid. *Lancet, 2*:983, 1963.
76. Norrell, H., and Wilson, C.: Brain tumor chemotherapy with methotrexate given intrathecally. *JAMA, 201*:15, 1967.

77. Ommaya, A.K., Rubin, R.C., Henderson, E.S., et al.: A new approach to the treatment of inoperable brain tumors. *Med Ann DC, 34*:455, 1965.
78. Rubin, R.C., Larson, R., and Rall, D.P.: 8-Azaguanine (NSC-749). I. Preclinical toxicity studies and a preliminary report on intrathecal perfusion therapy for patients. *Cancer Chemother Rep, 50*:283, 1966.
79. Rubin, R.C., Ommaya, A.K., Henderson, E.S., et al.: Cerebrospinal fluid perfusion for central nervous system neoplasms. *Neurology (Minneap), 16*:680, 1966.
80. Saiki, J.H., Thompson, S., Smith, F., and Atkinson, R.: Paraplegia following intrathecal chemotherapy. *Cancer, 29*:370, 1972.
81. Baum, E.S., Koch, H.F., Cordy, D.G., and Plunket, D.C.: Intrathecal methotrexate. *Lancet, 1*:649, 1971.
82. Bunge, R.P., and Settlage, P.H.: Neurological lesions in cats following cerebrospinal fluid manipulation. *J Neuropath Exp Neurol, 16*:471, 1957.
83. Lloyd, J.W., Hughes, J.T., and Davies-Jones, G.A.B.: Relief of severe intractable pain by barbotage of cerebrospinal fluid. *Lancet, 1*:354, 1972.
84. Bering, E.A., Jr., Wilson, C.B., and Norrell, H.A., Jr.: The Kentucky conference on brain tumor chemotherapy. *J Neurosurg, 27*:1, 1967.
85. Ringkjob, R.: Treatment of intracranial gliomas and metastatic carcinomas by local application of cytostatic agents. *Acta Neurol Scand, 44*:318, 1968.
86. Weiss, S.R., and Raskind, R.: Pathologic findings in brain tumors treated with local methotrexate. Unpublished observations.
87. Garfield, J., and Dayan, A.D.: Postoperative intracavitary chemotherapy of malignant gliomas. *J Neurosurg, 39*:315, 1973.
88. Bruce, W.R., Meeker, B.E., and Valeriote, F.: Comparison of the sensitivity of normal hematopoietic and transplanted lymphoma colony-forming cells to chemotherapeutic agents administered *in vivo. J Natl Cancer Inst, 37*:233, 1966.
89. Skipper, H.E., Schabel, F.M., Jr., Mellett, L.B., et al.: Implications of biochemical, cytokinetic, pharmacologic, and toxicologic relationships in the design of optimal therapeutic schedules. *Cancer Chemother Rep, 54*:431, 1970.

CHAPTER FOUR

EXPERIMENTAL
CHEMOTHERAPY MODELS

MARVIN BARKER

CHEMOTHERAPY OF MALIGNANT solid tumors will benefit considerably by the development of a reliable method for drug selection. Rapid tumor growth and toxicity caused by one or more unsuccessful courses of chemotherapy restrict the number of agents which can be given to a patient in a clinical trial. General experience indicates that many human tumors respond, at least temporarily, to a course of chemotherapy, despite their seeming development of resistance to an agent's effects. If an effective agent could be selected initially, the period of tumor inhibition could be prolonged by substituting a second and a third effective agent when drug resistance becomes apparent.

Rational chemotherapy of brain tumors should be based on an *in vitro* or animal model for determining a given tumor's sensitivity to a spectrum of chemotherapeutic agents.

IN VITRO MODELS

An *in vitro* test of tumor sensitivity to drugs would, in theory, be comparable to a bacteriological sensitivity test. A variety of such tests have been used for analyzing drug effectiveness against many types of human cancers, but only a few tests have been adaptable to brain tumors.

Murray, et al.[1] employed a double coverslip lying-drop culture, adding the test compound to the medium, which was renewed four times over a ten day observation period. The degree of cell damage was rated according to: (1) inhibition of cell migration, (2) inhibition of mitosis, (3) nuclear changes, (4) cytoplasmic changes, and (5) blunting of cell processes and rounding of cells. Using 8-azaguanine, Murray and coworkers observed progres-

75

sively severe damage which was lethal within ten days for most tumors tested. However, responses to the test agent varied among different areas and tissue types within the same tumor. The response of similar tumors from different individuals also varied.

Walker and Wright[2] reported that vinblastine sulfate produced a wide range of cytologic alterations in primary cultures of human neoplasms. However, only one glial tumor, a glioblastoma, was included in their assay.

Easty and Wylie[3] assayed the sensitivity of various cultured brain tumors to several drugs using cultivated HeLa cells as controls. No consistent differences in sensitivity were observed among the cell cultures, although cytotoxicity varied widely among the different drugs: methotrexate was inactive in this system; melphalan and chlorambucil acted rapidly, but ultimately proved less toxic than Thiotepa; and, although vinblastine sulfate was found to be highly cytotoxic, its effect on cells *in vitro* was nevertheless variable.

Gazso and Afra[4] investigated the cytostatic effects of two antibiotics, actinomycin C and actinomycin D, on cultures of glioblastomas, astrocytomas, and meningiomas. The results were quantified and compared by determining the growth inhibition rates and the mitotic indices of the explants; qualitatively, alterations in cell morphology were evaluated.

Mealey, et al.[5] found that the cytotoxicity of mithramycin and vincristine against eight malignant gliomas *in vitro* differed from the cytotoxic effect that had been assumed on the bases of clinical responses in patients harboring the neoplasms. Qualitative cytomorphologic assessment demonstrated variable sensitivity among cultures of glioblastoma derived from different patients and treated with different doses, but virtually all cultures showed some susceptibility, ranging from slight to extreme, to both drugs.

Technique for Drug Sensitivity Studies

The author has conducted extensive drug sensitivity studies using the method described below.

Leighton tubes containing flying coverslips were prepared as primary explant cultures, or prepared by trypsinization of older monolayer cultures grown by a method the author used for several years.[6,8] Potential oncolytic agents were added during the culture's proliferative phase — on the eighth day in primary cultures, and after twenty-four hours in established cultures. Drug contact with the cells varied in duration from three to four days. Drug concentrations ranged from 1×10^{-5} to 5,120 mcg/cc, except if a particular agent's solubility limited such high concentrations. At the end of the chosen contact time, the medium was removed and the coverslip culture was washed in balanced salt solution, fixed in methanol and stained with Giemsa's stain.

The extent of cell-kill was the basis for rating drug results. Originally the author determined two end points for drug toxicity, the lethal end point (LE); and the cytotoxic end point (CE). The LE was the concentration of drug at which target cells were completely lysed; the CE expressed the drug concentration that produced morphologic change in at least 75 percent of target cells.

Vinblastine. The author first tested vinblastine sulfate against an established tumor cell line (TC 34, a glioblastoma) to ascertain the optimal age of cultures for drug addition. When the drug was added immediately after cell transferral, cytotoxic effects as well as growth inhibition resulted. A clearer end point was obtained when the drug was not added until at least twenty-four hours after transfer; during this interval the cells attached to the surface of the culture vessel and entered an active growth phase.

In fourteen cultures treated with vinblastine sulfate, LE values for five glioblastomas ranged from 50 to 500 mcg/cc, and CE values ranged from 5×10^{-3} to 5×10^{-5} mcg/cc. An ependymoma and normal astrocytes from both guinea pig and human were relatively resistant to vinblastine sulfate; in three astrocytomas, a mixed glioma, a meningioma, and a neuroblastoma, LE values were equal to or lower than those for glioblastomas. Repeat studies on the same tumors resulted in identical LE's, while the CE's varied somewhat. These variations depended on the culture's age when the drug was added and on the duration of drug/cell contact.

In contrast, the LE's did not deviate under different drug

schedules or with varying culture ages. The LE's were more easily determined than CE's, because the latter required microscopic separation of normal from abnormal cells. In all instances, cytologic abnormalities were detected from one to two hours after vinblastine had been added to the cultures. Abnormalities included: increased cytoplasmic density, poor staining of cytoplasmic membranes, cytoplasmic vaculization, nuclear pyknosis, multinucleation, fusion of nuclei within multinucleated cells, and conglomeration of damaged cells.[9]

Vincristine sulfate, nitrogen mustard, and phenylalanine mustard were assayed in similar brain tumor cultures, using the technique described above. Although these agents were as toxic as vinblastine sulfate had been, they were not studied further because their value in clinical chemotherapy of brain tumors has proved to be limited.

Mithramycin. Mithramycin assays in numerous cultured brain tumors produced endpoints and morphologic changes that compared favorably with those of vinblastine sulfate in the same type of cultures. Cytotoxic concentrations ranged from 0.0006 to 5.0 mcg/cc with vinblastine and from 0.08 to 40 mcg/cc with mithramycin. Lethal end point concentrations ranged from 2.5 to 5,120 mcg/cc with vinblastine and from 0.15 to more than 5,120 mcg/cc with mithramycin. Patterns of sensitivity could not be correlated with tumor type or culture age.

When brain tumor cells were exposed to mithramycin, cytoplastic membranes contracted, and at higher concentrations, cytoplasm disintegrated into irregularly shaped globules and strands. Mithramycin induced pronounced alterations in nuclear sizes and shapes and even more striking changes in amount and deposition of nuclear chromatin.[10]

Culture Media Studies. The effect of a given culture medium on vinblastine sulfate and mithramycin toxicity in brain tumors was then studied. Media used were Puck's N-16 medium and human cerebrospinal fluid, the latter having been proved an excellent medium for culturing brain tumors.[7] In ten experiments, lethal concentrations were identical, and in two experiments, concentrations differed by four dilutions. Cytotoxic endpoints in Puck's medium and in CSF were identical in three experiments, and in the remainder, differences ranged from one to three dilutions. Again, no pattern of relative sensitivity could be correlated with a specific drug, tumor type, or culture age.[11]

Hydrocortisone. Tricyanoaminopropene and hydrocortisone, although unrelated chemically and differing from each other in mechanisms of action, exerted similar effects on brain tumor cultures. At drug concentrations below cytotoxic levels, both agents stimulated growth, an effect never observed with the agents described previously. At high concentrations, the drugs had a direct cytotoxic action, and inhibited the growth of tumor cell cultures.[8]

Methotrexate. Experiments with methotrexate, an antimetabolite, failed because the medium used for culturing brain tumors contains folic acid. Although some morphologic changes and growth inhibition occurred at high concentrations, a lethal effect was never observed.[8]

BCNU. The alkylating agent, 1,3-bis-(2-chloroethyl)-1-nitrosourea (BCNU) had shown oncolytic activity in diverse human solid tumors before it had been suggested as a possible brain tumor chemotherapeutic agent. The ability of BCNU to rapidly cross the intact blood-brain barrier prompted its use in extensive experimental and clinical trials. The author conducted eighteen experiments with BCNU in nine cultured brain tumors, ranging in age from twenty-five to 2425 days. Lethal endpoint values of vinblastine sulfate had been determined in many of the same tumors. BCNU's LE values ranged from 80 to 640 mcg/cc, while vinblastine's LE values ranged from 160 to 640 mcg/cc. Drug sensitivity could not be correlated with tumor type or with culture age. Cytotoxic effects of BCNU, as judged by morphologic abnormalities, were apparent with concentrations as low as 20 mcg/cc. The morphologic changes were identical to those produced by vinblastine.

Only LE values were determined for BCNU since, by this time in his studies, the author had not developed the value of determining the CE. The objective of chemotherapy is irreversible damage or tumor cell death. To examine the relationship between cytotoxic alterations and tumor viability, he used vital staining as an indication of cell death. It was found that many cells remained viable despite the extent of morphologic change. He concluded that the CE was not a valid criterion of drug sensitivity, and that complete cytolysis (LE) was more relevant in clinical applications of oncolytic agents.

Evaluation of Method

Figure 4-1 summarizes the characteristic responses of cultured brain tumors to all chemotherapeutic agents investigated. An analysis of the *in vitro* testing method for drug sensitivity produced three major limitations to the applicability of *in vitro* data to clinical chemotherapy: (1) A drug's concentration at the LE is far higher than its systemically toxic dose; (2) A drug's observed LE does not necessarily result from the drug's principal oncolytic action, but may be due to side-effects produced by high concentrations of the drug; and (3) End points are derived in an artificial environment and cannot be correlated with drug effect *in vivo* because normal neuroglia proliferate in cell culture at a rate comparable to that of neoplastic neuroglia. Therefore, there is no system for determining relative degrees of *in vitro* drug sensitivity, i.e., a therapeutic index.

On the other hand, encouraging data indicates that a drug, BCNU, with which the author has obtained excellent results in clinical trials and in experimental animal models, also has marked cytotoxic effects on brain tumor cells *in vitro*.

Interest in cell cultures for testing drugs has been renewed by recent information concerning the kinetic characteristics of human gliomas. The author has always used target cells during their proliferative or log phase growth. When cultured tumor cells enter a stationary phase of growth they present growth patterns similar to those of tumors, *in vivo*; for example, because of overcrowding and lack of nutrients, cells enter a nonproliferating phase and LI and GF fall to low values. When tumor cells are cultured in a rich medium they tend to dedifferentiate rapidly, with proliferation becoming their sole function. A poor medium, which provides only basic nutrients, slows growth, and to some extent, retards dedifferentiation, presents a more appropriate system for chemotherapy assays.

The author also used gross methods to determine drug toxicity.

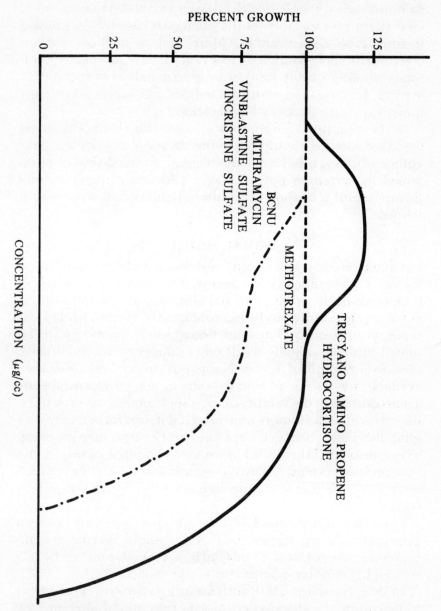

Figure 4-1. Diagram illustrating the characteristic responses of glial cell cultures to various oncolytic agents.

Percent growth = cells in treated culture

cells in control culture x 100

(Modified from Wilson and Barker [8])

As noted earlier, the CE described is not a valid therapeutic index; vital stains give variable results when cells have firmly attached themselves to a glass surface. More accurate methods, such as determination of plating efficiency, of LI, or of rate of DNA synthesis would probably yield more precise indices of therapeutic activity. Investigation of these methods and others is currently underway in the author's laboratories.

In the meantime, reservations as noted concerning the above-described method should be a consideration in evaluating the author's findings; however, the method outlined should be retained for screening potential agents for brain tumor chemotherapy, until a method of greater reliability and sensitivity is refined.

ANIMAL MODELS

Animal models have been used extensively for preclinical testing of chemotherapeutic agents. The numbers and kinds of tumors available in experimental animals are virtually infinite. Some are chemically produced or induced by viruses, while some occur spontaneously. The induction of some tumors requires an inbred strain of animals, while other tumors are transplantable, even in a noninbred strain. Numerous models have also been available for testing potential brain tumor chemotherapeutic agents, although the validity of most such models has been questioned because the tumors were nonglial in origin, or if they were glial, the tumors had been implanted in sites other than the brain. The transplantability of brain tumors, regardless of origin, has been reviewed extensively by Wilson and Bates.[12] The author used several of these tumor systems as models for chemotherapy testing.

Intracerebral leukemia L1210 in mice has been used to screen potential oncolytic agents for C.N.S. (central nervous system) leukemia. Schabel, et al.[13] and Chirigos, et al.[14] found that BCNU was highly effective against this tumor model.

In 1965, Norrell and Wilson[15] conducted a series of experiments to determine the effectiveness of I.T. injection of methotrexate against transplanted brain tumors in rats. Mean survival was 12.6 days for rats bearing tumors transplanted from a human oligodendroglioma grown in cell culture. Mean survival was 14.1 days for animals receiving methotrexate I.P. The mean survival was 17.0 days for rats bearing the same tumor but receiving methotrexate intracisternally. Enhanced drug effect after intracisternal administration was attributed to methotrexate's limited penetration of the blood-brain barrier.

Another model used by Wilson, et al.[16] was the penetration of uniform intracerebral tumors in rats by transplanting a methylcholanthrene-induced rat mammary sarcoma from cell culture. Control rats bearing these tumors survived a mean of 18.0 days. Experimental animals treated with I.P. methotrexate survived a mean of 19.1 days, while those treated intracisternally survived a mean of 18.9 days. Using the same tumor model, Wilson's group found that vinblastine sulfate infused via the common carotid artery increased average survival from 15.2 to 15.6 days. Intraperitoneal vinblastine injection increased survival to 16.8 days when the tumor model was modified by implanting tumors in both cerebral hemispheres; untreated animals survived an average of only 12.5 days. Infusion of methotrexate via the common carotid artery over forty-eight hours decreased average survivial to 12.1 days. Intraperitoneal injection raised average survival to 14.3 days, while intracisternal injections proved the most effective drug route, increasing average survival to 15.8 days.

Kotsilimbas, et al.[17,18] used a melanoma transplanted to mouse brain as a model for testing corticosteroids and parenteral 5-FU against brain tumors. Although Donelli, et al.[19,20] and Wright and coworkers[21] used glial tumors, they transplanted the tumor to the animal's flank in their chemotherapy model.

Intracerebral Glial Tumor Models

An attempt to test chemotherapeutic agents against a glial tumor implanted in animal brain was first reported by Ausman, Shapiro, and Slivka, in 1968.[22] This model was based on the carcinogen-induced murine ependymoblastoma. Zimmerman and Arnold,[23] Seligman and Shear,[24] and Sigiura[25] all used models employing a chemically-induced ependymoblastoma but differing in several biological characteristics. Fragments of subcutaneously-carried tumors were implanted into the brains of mice by a technique that permitted preparation of many animals in a short time. The tumors grew and proved fatal in a predictable interval. Animals lost weight and developed central nervous system signs (e.g., spinning, limb paralysis) about five days before death. These mice could be treated with chemotherapeutic agents under controlled circumstances and any increased life span could be determined.

This murine glioma model has been used to test the following drugs: (1) BCNU, (2) cyclophosphamide, (3) mithramycin, (4) methotrexate, (5) CCNU, (6) vincristine, and (7) 5-fluorouracil.[22,26,30].

BCNU was highly effective against three strains of murine glioma. The increased life span over controls varied from 31 to 38 percent, and up to 35 percent of treated animals were long-term survivors (beyond sixty days). Cyclophosphamide was also effective, but survival time over controls rarely exceeded 30 percent. Both drugs were given I.P. as a single injection. Mithramycin was ineffective on a single-injection schedule as well as a five-day schedule in doses that ranged from $L.D._0$ to $L.D._{100}$. Methotrexate, given every four days in four doses, did not significantly increase life span. CCNU was effective when administered up to two weeks following tumor implantation, although the number of long-term survivors decreased with progressively delayed therapy. Vincristine and 5-FU failed to increase survival.

The murine glioma of Shapiro, et al. provides an excellent model for testing potential oncolytic agents in the therapy of brain tumors. However, this particular model fails to satisfy all criteria for an ideal brain tumor model: (1) The tumor should be a primary brain tumor; (2) The tumor should be transplantable to the animal brain; (3) The tumor take should be predictable and reproducible; (4) The survival span should be long enough to permit therapy well after the implantation procedure; and (5) The host animal should be suitable for all clinical routes of therapy. In the ependymoblastoma the tumor cell types are heterogeneous and the tumor behaves more like a metastatic than a primary tumor. In addition, the use of tumor fragments, where small differences in size and viability may exist, leads to a wide range of survival.

The author's laboratory uses three mouse glioma models. The ependymoblastoma, glioma 26, and glioma 261, as described by Ausman, et al.,[27] are maintained in cell culture. Instead of solid tumor fragments, trypsinized single cell suspensions of these tumor cells are injected intracerebrally with a repeating dispenser syringe delivering 4×10^4 cells in 10μl. A 25 or 27 gauge short bevel needle with a stop at 3 mm provides consistent tumor placement. These models are used mainly for screening potential oncolytic agents.

New Rat Brain Tumor Model

The author has developed a new animal model for brain tumors.[31] The tumor was induced in CD Fisher rats by weekly intravenous injections of N-nitrosomethylurea. Tissue culture and preservation methods have been described by Benda, et al.[32] In the laboratory, these cells are grown in Eagle's Basal Medium®, supplemented with 10 percent fetal calf serum, excess L-glutamine and antibiotics, by the monolayer method for continuous cell culture described previously.[6] Adequate numbers of cells are preserved in liquid nitrogen to insure against loss of the cell line. The morphology of the tumor in cell culture is similar to that of cultured human astrocytomas.

Transplantation. The procedure for transplantation of cultured cells to rat brain is as follows: Forty-eight hour cultures are harvested by trypsinization and adjusted to a concentration of 4×10^6 cells in Gey's balanced salt solution. Adult male CD Fisher rats are anesthetized and placed in a small-animal stereotaxic head holder. The scalp is opened electrosurgically and a 0.07-inch hole is drilled at a point 2.5 mm to the left of the midline and 4.0 mm anterior to the frontal zero plane according to Koenig's Atlas.[33] The hole is plugged with a stainless steel screw (0.125 x 0.0625 inch) having a 0.0292 inch center-drilled hole. The cell suspension (0.01 cc) is injected into the central white matter through a blunt 22 gauge needle attached to a 0.1 cc chromatography syringe, with the needle extending 3.0 mm beyond the tip of the screw. The central screw hole is immediately sealed with bone wax to prevent reflux, and the scalp incision is closed with a skin clip.

Death in these animals is preceded by a predictable period of symptoms lasting five to six days: (1) weight loss of 5 to 10 gm daily, (2) increased tear secretion and red pigmentation around the eyes, (3) paresis (progressing to paralysis) starting in the right side and becoming bilateral, involving the hindlegs first and not always appearing in the forelegs, and (4) generalized convulsions. Caudal displacement of the brain causes death.

Intracerebral tumor was present in all animals; in a few, subdural and subcutaneous spread of tumor occurred from leakage of the cell suspension during injection. The tumor is greyish, well circumscribed, and firmer than the surrounding brain. It is detectable microscopically after seven to ten days and macroscopically by the fourteenth day. Lethal tumors are five to seven mm in diameter and weight approximately 200 mg.

The percentage of tumor takes has been 100 percent in all control experiments. The median survival of control animals has varied from twenty-two to thirty-five days in different experiments, but the range of survival in each experimental group has been within acceptable limits.

Histological Change. The histology of the original tumor was that of an astrocytoma with anaplastic features.[34] After approximately six months in cell culture, the tumor produced intracerebrally presented a different morphology. This change was gradual; after continuous culture for 2.5 years, the tumor produced after intercerebral transplantation was well circumscribed but not encapsulated, and although similar to the original tumor, it contained bizarre nuclear forms and more zones of necrosis surrounded by palisading tumor cells. Staining with PTAH demonstrated the glial nature of this portion of the tumor, although extracellular fibers stained poorly. In addition to this glial component there were, coursing through the tumor, interdigitating bundles of spindle cells that had vesicular, elongated nuclei with more prominent nucleoli. These cells showed less pleomorphism than those of the glial component, and were associated with abundant reticulin and considerable collagen production. Mitoses were observed in this component, although less frequently than in the glial component. The profound desmoplastic response exceeded the limits of a purely reactive process and was best interpreted as being neoplastic on the basis of histologic features. The presence of the two distinct cell types dictated reclassification as a gliosarcoma.

The longer the tumor remained in continuous culture, the longer the median survival time of each experimental group. The early cultures produced a lethal tumor in approximately twenty-two days, and although the tumor cell inoculum remained constant (4 x 10^6/cc), after continuous culture for two years the median survival time increased to thirty-five days. When banked primary explant cultures were returned to cell culture and then used for implantation, no evidence was seen of morphological change, and median survival time returned to approximately twenty-two days.

Advantages. The tumor used in this experimental system satisfies the first criterion of a primary brain tumor. The tumors resulting from implantation of cultured cells remained typical astrocytomas until sarcomatous transformation was noted after six months of continuous culture. Unfortunately, the author has been unable to eliminate the sarcomatous element by cloning; and while this does lessen the purity of the model, he feels it does not impose undue limitations on its use.

The ease with which the tumor can be transplanted to the brain satisfies one of the major criteria for an animal model. The reproducibility of the model (100%) was surprising, since there is a low frequency of "no take" even in the best of systems. The median survival span among different experiments varied, probably because of mechanical errors such as cell count, viability of the cells, and size of the rats, but the range of survival was acceptable within each experimental group. Therefore, with an adequate number of tumor-bearing control animals, the probability of detecting an effective chemotherapeutic agent in this system is high. The survival time of more than twenty days allows the administration of drugs well after the immediate postimplantation period. A major advantage of this particular model is an animal large enough to permit alternative routes of drug administration, e.g. intrathecal[16] and arterial injection or infusion.[15]

Rat Model Drug Assays

BCNU. This model as described has been used to assay several chemotherapeutic agents. For two reasons BCNU was the first drug tested: first, BCNU had shown activity in patients harboring primary brain tumors; and second, the effect of BCNU against intracerebral L1210 leukemia tumors and mouse gliomas had been reported. Five experiments were carried out using two doses of BCNU administered by two different schedules. Equal numbers of tumor-bearing rats were randomly selected for nontreated controls and treated animals. Either a 40 percent $L.D._{10}$ or an 80 percent $L.D._{10}$ dose of BCNU was administered I.P. on days nine and sixteen postimplantation or on days sixteen and twenty-three postimplantation.

The results (shown in Table 4-I) indicated that BCNU, when given in tolerated doses by an I.P. route, not only increased the survival of rats bearing intracerebral gliomas when given on days nine and sixteen (38% to 84%), but also produced a significantly increased lifespan when treatment was delayed until the sixteenth and twenty-third days (41% to 75%). This increased survival with delayed treatment was observed even in those experiments where untreated rats were already showing symptoms. These results not only confirmed the findings of Schabel, et al.[13] Chirigos, et al.[14] and Shapiro, et al.[26,30] but also indicated that BCNU is effective against older, larger tumors that contain a high proportion of nonproliferating cells.

Four animals in BCNU-treated groups were still alive at 98, 185, 185, and 275 days after tumor transplantation. These animals were killed and autopsy revealed no tumor. Of course, there is the possibility that these were simply cases of no-take tumors, but it seems highly unlikely that no-takes should occur in two closely related experiments when the animal model has been established hundreds of times previously with death in 100% of control and treated animals. It is also highly unlikely that all four no-take animals should be in treated groups when randomization of tumor-bearing animals before treatment was a standard procedure.

A morphological comparison of tumors removed from the

TABLE 4-I*

Statistical analysis of effect of BCNU on survival of rats bearing brain tumors
All BCNU-treated animals received 80% of an LD_{10}, unless otherwise indicated.

Experimental group	No. of animals	Survival time (days)		Median survival (days)	Range (days)	ILS (%)	p
1. Control	8	24.5	3.16	25	8		
BCNU	8	37	11.3	34.5	20	38	0.0001
BCNU	6	46	17.4	46	45	84	0.0001
2. Control	10	29.1	4.72	28	14		
BCNU	12	40	6.89	40.5	23	41	0.0001
3. Control	12	29.75	6.56	28	25		
BCNU	12	39.75	7.4	39.5	25	41	0.0001
4. Control	10	35.8	7.64	36.5	25		
BCNU	8	66	19	64	56	75	0.0001
5. Control	10	37.4	4.76	36	15		
BCNU	10	55.3	10.7	53	36	47	0.0001

Determined by Wilcoxon rank sum test.
Received 40% of an LD .
Mean   S.D.

*(Reprinted from Barker, et al., reference 31, with permission of the publisher.)

brains of treated and untreated animals at death produced two striking observations. The cellular morphology presented by treated tumors was quite similar to that found when cell cultures of the rat glioma were exposed to graded concentrations of BCNU. This same type of cellular morphology was observed in cell cultures of tumors removed from patients subsequent to BCNU therapy. Another feature of BCNU-treated rat gliomas was extensive necrosis. Comparable necrosis was never observed in untreated tumors, and the numerous foci of necrosis were attributed to cell death as a result of BCNU therapy.

Corticosteroids. This animal model has also been used to investigate the antitumor effect of corticosteroids. Gurcay, et al.[35,36] have shown that methylprednisolone acetate given on the tenth, thirteenth, and nineteenth days postimplantation reduced the weight of tumors removed on day twenty-one from an average weight of 157.5 mg to an average weight of 36.25 mg. Control animals in a second experiment survived an average of 28.7 days; corticosteroid-treated animals survived an average of 37.4 days.

Irradiation. In the laboratory the effect of irradiation with and without concurrent BCNU therapy produced the following results. BCNU (80% of L.D.$_{10}$) was administered on days sixteen and twenty-three and irradiation (400 r) was given daily from day sixteen through day twenty-six. Average survival times were as follows.

Control rats	35.8 days
Irradiated rats	49.9 days
BCNU-treated rats	60.7 days
Irradiated-BCNU-	
treated rats	62.3 days

Other therapy trials involved: (1) CCNU, orally and I.P. which proved to be as effective as BCNU, (2) vincristine sulfate, which did not extend survival, and (3) L-asparaginase, which did not extend survival.

Tumor Model Kinetics

After analyzing the results of these experiments, the author reasoned that knowledge of the growth kinetics of this tumor system should provide a basis for selecting drugs and designing drug schedules. Recent advances in the treatment of leukemia have resulted directly from studies in an animal model of great predictive value,[37] and the majority of data on tumor cell kinetics has been obtained using this and similar animal models. However, information from these models is not applicable to intracerebral tumors. The few reports of *in vivo* studies of human glioblastomas have been based on calculations made using assumed DNA synthesis times.[38, 40] Recent work from the author's laboratory on the kinetics of human brain tumors *in vivo* provided a stimulus to define the kinetic parameters of the animal model.[41,42]

In cell culture the proliferation characteristics of rat glioma cells varied according to the quantity of nutrients in the medium and the available surface area. Tumor cells grew exponentially to a population of 1.5 million cells per 3-oz prescription bottle (available growth area = 30 cm²). If the medium was not changed, the population became stationary. Replacing one-half of the medium each day permitted growth to a population of 15 million cells per 3-oz bottle. At this population density, the available space was covered with tightly packed cells, and a stationary phase appeared briefly. Then cell death, evidenced by peeling of the monolayer and accumulation of cell debris in the medium, led to an abrupt decrease in the cell population to 1.5 million cells per bottle. One-half of the medium was then replaced each day, and the population gradually increased again to 15 million cells. Thus, the growth pattern of these cultures could be classified in three categories: (1) cells in exponential growth, (2) cells in a stationary phase due to starvation, and (3) cells with variable proliferation due to overcrowding and repopulation.

The kinetic parameters of the rat glioma could not be determined during the earliest stages of tumor growth, since tumor cells were only rarely identified before the twelfth day postimplantation. Therefore, the calculated kinetic parameters are those of a tumor in the late stages of proliferation immediately before the onset of symptoms in the animal host. The parameters obtained for the rat glioma *in vivo* were:[31]

cell cycle time (Tc)	= 20 hrs
DNA synthesis (Ts)	= 10 hours
mitotic period (Tm)	= 1 to 2 hrs.
G1 Phase (T_{G1})	= 6 to 7 hrs
G2 Phase (T_{G2})	= 2 to 2.5 hrs
labeling index (LI)	= 15 to 20%
growth fraction (GF)	= 0.35 to 0.46
observed doubling time (Td)	= 72 hrs
cell loss factor (CLF)	= 0.42

The long doubling time and the high cell loss factor indicate that this tumor is comparable to the human brain tumor.

Information concerning cell population kinetics should provide a more rational basis for the design of drug schedules in brain tumor chemotherapy. This is true not only for phase-dependent drugs, but also for drug combinations, e.g. a cell cycle-nonspecific drug like BCNU and a cell cycle-phase-specific drug like vincristine sulfate.[43, 44] For example, vincristine sulfate could be scheduled so that it arrested proliferating cycling cells during intervals between BCNU. Combination chemotherapy can be applied to the rat model, and, with additional knowledge of the kinetic parameters of human gliomas, schedules successful in the laboratory can be translated into clinical chemotherapy.

This animal model has proven to be as reliable as other brain tumor models in assaying drug effectiveness, and as it offers some advantages over other models, it should fulfill the needs of experimental chemotherapists. Not only can the model be used for screening of unknown oncolytic agents, but also, with the added knowledge of its growth patterns, it can be used to develop optimal dosage schedules for new drugs and combined modality protocols.

REFERENCES

1. Murray, M.R., Peterson, E.R., Hirschberg, E., and Pool, J.L.: Metabolic and chemotherapeutic investigation of human glioblastoma *in vitro. Ann NY Acad Sci, 58*:1147, 1954.

2. Walker, D.G. and Wright, J.C.: The effect of vincaleukoblastine on primary cultures of human neoplasms. A preliminary report. *Cancer Chemother Rep, 14*:139, 1961.

3. Easty, D.M. and Wylie, J.A.: Screening of 12 gliomata against chemotherapeutic agents *in vitro. Br Med J, 5345*:1589, 1963.

4. Gazso, L.R. and Afra, D.: Study on the effect of actinomycins in tissue cultures from human brain tumors. *Acta Neurochir (Wien), 21*:139, 1969.

5. Mealey, J., Jr., Chen, T.T., and Pedlow, E.: Brain tumor chemotherapy with mithramycin and vincristine. *Cancer, 26*:360, 1970.

6. Wilson, C.B., Barker, M., and Slagel, D.E.: Tumors of the central nervous system in monolayer tissue. *Arch Neurol, 15*:275, 1966.

7. Wilson, C.B. and Barker, M.: Cerebrospinal fluid as a culture medium for human brain tumors. *Neurology (Minneap), 16*:1064, 1966.

8. Wilson, C.B. and Barker, M.: Studies of malignant brain tumors in cell culture. *Ann NY Acad Sci, 159*:480, 1969.

9. Wilson, C.B. and Barker, M.: Sensitivity of cell cultures of neural tumors to vinblastine sulfate (NSC-49842). *Cancer Chemother Rep, 44*:9, 1965.

10. Wilson, C.B. and Barker, M.: Relative cytotoxicity of mithramycin and vinblastine sulfate in cell cultures of human neural tumors. *J Natl Cancer Inst, 38*:459, 1967.

11. Wilson, C.B. and Barker, M.: Chemotherapeutic response of human glial tumor cells cultured in cerebrospinal fluid. *Cancer Chemother Rep, 51*:201, 1967.

12. Wilson, Charles B. and Bates, Ernest A.: Transplantable brain tumors. In Kirsch, Wolff M., Grossi Paoletti, Enrica, and Paoletti, Pietro (Eds.): *The Experimental Biology of Brain Tumors.* Springfield, Thomas, 1972, pp. 19-56.

13. Schabel, F.M., Jr., Johnston, T.P., McCaleb, G.S., et al.: Experimental evaluation of potential anticancer agents. VIII. Effects of certain nitrosoureas on intracerebral L1210 leukemia. *Cancer Res, 23*:725, 1963.

14. Chirigos, M.A., Humphreys, S.R., and Goldin, A.: Duration of effective levels of three antitumor drugs in mice with leukemia L1210 implanted intracerebrally and subcutaneously. *Cancer Chemother Rep, 49*:15, 1965.

15. Norrell, H.A. and Wilson, C.B.: Chemotherapy of experimental brain tumors by arterial infusion. *Surg Forum, 16*:429, 1965.

16. Wilson, C.B., Norell, H., Jr., and Barker, M.: Intrathecal injection of methotrexate (NSC-740) in transplanted brain tumors. *Cancer Chemother Rep, 51*:1, 1967.

17. Kotsilimbas, D.G., Karpf, R., Meredith S., and Scheinberg, L.C.: Evaluation of parenteral 5-FU on experimental brain tumors. *Neurology (Minneap), 16*:916, 1966.

18. Kotsilimbas, D.G., Meyer, L., Berson, M., et al.: Corticosteroid effect on intracerebral melanomata and associated cerebral edema. Some unexpected findings. *Neurology (Minneap), 17*:223, 1967.

19. Donelli, M.G., Rosso, R., and Garattini, S.: Selective chemotherapy in relation to the site of tumor transplantation. *Int J Cancer, 2*:421, 1967.

20. Rosso, R., Donelli, M.G., Reyers-Degli Innocenti, I., and Garattini, S.: Chemotherapy of tumors transplanted intracerebrally. *Eur J Cancer, 3*:125, 1967.

21. Wright, R.L., Shaumba, B., and Keller, J.: The effect of glucocorticosteroids on growth and metabolism of experimental glial tumors. *J Neurosurg, 30*:140, 1969.

22. Ausman, J.I., Shapiro, W.R., and Slivka, J.J.: The effect of chemotherapeutic agents on an experimental mouse brain tumor. *Proc Am Assoc Cancer Res, 9*:4, 1968.

23. Zimmerman, H.M. and Arnold, H.: Experimental brain tumors. I. Tumors produced with methylcholanthrene. *Cancer Res, 1*:919, 1941.

24. Seligman, A.M. and Shear, M.J.: Studies in carcinogenesis. VIII. Experimental production of brain tumors in mice with methylcholanthrene. *Am J Cancer, 37*:364, 1939.

25. Sugiura, K.: Tumor transplantation. In Gay, W.I., (Ed.): *Methods of Animal Experimentation*. New York, Acad Pr, 1969, vol. II, pp. 171-222.
26. Shapiro, W.R. and Ausman, J.I.: Effect of chemotherapeutic agents on experimental brain tumors. *Proc Am Assoc Cancer Res, 10:*79, 1969.
27. Ausman, J.I., Shapiro, W.R., and Rall, D.P.: Studies on the chemotherapy of experimental brain tumors: development of an experimental model. *Cancer Res, 30:*2394, 1970.
28. Levin, V.A., Shapiro, W.R., Clancy, T.P., and Oliverio, V.T.: The uptake, distribution, and antitumor activity of 1-(2-chloroethyl)-3-cyclohexyl-1-nitrosourea in the murine glioma. *Cancer Res, 30:*2451, 1970.
29. Shapiro, W.R., Ausman, J.I., and Rall, D.P.: Studies on the chemotherapy of experimental brain tumors: evaluation of 1,-3-bis(2-chloroethyl)-1-nitrosourea, cyclophosphamide, mithramycin and methotrexate. *Cancer Res, 30:*2401, 1970.
30. Shapiro, W.R.: Studies on the chemotherapy of experimental brain tumors: evaluation of 1-(2-chloroethyl)-3-cyclohexyl-1-nitrosourea, vincristine, and 5-fluorouracil. *J Natl Cancer Inst, 46:*359, 1971.
31. Barker, M., Hoshino, T., Gurcay, O., et al.: Development of an animal brain tumor model and its response to therapy with 1,3-bis(2-chloroethyl)-1-nitrosourea. *Cancer Res, 33:*976, 1973.
32. Benda, P., Someda, K., Messer, J., and Sweet, W.H..: Morphological and immunochemical studies of rat glial tumors and clonal strains propagated in culture. *J Neurosurg, 34:*310, 1971.
33. Konig, J.F.R. and Klippel, R.A.: *The Rat Brain: A Stereotaxic Atlas of the Forebrain and Lower Parts of the Brain Stem*. Baltimore, Williams & Wilkins, 1963.
34. Schmidek, H.A., Nielsen, S.L., Schiller, A.L., and Messer, J.: Morphological studies of rat brain tumors induced by N-nitrosomethylurea. *J Neurosurg, 34:*335, 1971.
35. Gurcay, O., Wilson, C.B., and Eliason, J.: The effect of methylprednisolone acetate on transplantable rat glioma. *Surg Forum, 21:*437, 1970.
36. Gurcay, O., Wilson, C.B., Barker, M., and Eliason, J.: Corticosteroid effect on transplantable rat glioma. *Arch Neurol, 24:*266, 1971.
37. Young, R.C. and DeVita, V.T.: The effect of chemotherapy on the growth characteristics and cellular kinetics of leukemia L1210. *Cancer Res, 30:*1789, 1970.
38. Johnson, H.A., Haymaker, W.E., Rubini, J.R., et al.: A radiographic study of a human brain and glioblastoma multiforme after the *in vivo* uptake of triated thymidine. *Cancer, 13:*636, 1960.
39. Tym, R.: Distribution of cell doubling times in in vivo human cerebral tumors. *Surg Forum, 20:*445, 1969.
40. Fukuma, S., Taketomo, S., Ueda, S., et al.: Autoradiographic studies of the growth of brain tumors using local labeling with ^{3}H-thymidine *in vivo*. *Brain Nerve, 21:*1029, 1969.
41. Hoshino, T., Barker, M., Wilson, C.B., et al.: Cell kinetics of human

gliomas. *J Neurosurg, 37*:15, 1972.

42. Wilson, C.B., Hoshino, T., Barker, M., and Downey, R.: Kinetics of gliomas in rat and man. In Bingham, W.G., Jr. (Ed.): *Recent Advances in Brain Tumor Research, (Progress in Experimental Tumor Research, Vol. 17).* Basel, Karger, 1972, pp. 363-372.

43. Rall, D.P. and Homan, E.R.: Possible approaches in selective toxicity: new concepts in cancer chemotherapy. *Cancer Chemother Rep, 51*:247, 1967.

44. Schatel, M., Jr.: Personal communication.

CHAPTER FIVE

PATIENT SELECTION
AND EVALUATION

DEREK FEWER AND CHARLES B. WILSON

BASIC RESEARCH, INCLUDING cell kinetics and other behavior observed in experimental tumors, must ultimately culminate in clinical application. Brain tumor chemotherapy is a relatively new treatment modality and it has thus far employed agents still undergoing clinical trials in rigidly defined Phase Studies.

This chapter details the nature of and patient selection for the three clinical phases and criteria for ascertaining the clinical response to drugs under study. These points are important for those who may wish to design their own studies of oncolytic agents for brain tumors.

SELECTION OF PATIENTS

Phase I

A Phase I trial establishes the maximum tolerated dose of a drug and its optimum schedule and route of administration. This is done by determining the limiting toxicity (e.g., bone-marrow depression, gastrointestinal ulceration) and the degree to which this toxicity is reversible. Such a study involves the administration of drugs to patients with advanced cancer unresponsive to conventional therapy.

Because documentation of antitumor effectiveness is not an objective in Phase I trials, patients with nonmeasurable tumor masses may be included. For ethical reasons, only patients with end-stage cancer of any type who have already received all forms of standard treatment (including chemotherapy) should be accepted for a Phase I study. However, patients with a brief life expectancy are not suitable candidates, since a follow-up period of eight weeks is usually required to detect dose-limiting toxicity from even a single treatment. Because the majority of oncolytic drugs affect bone marrow, patients with neoplastic involvement of bone marrow and depleted bone marrow reserve from previous chemotherapy should be excluded, and the patient's kidneys, liver, and cardiovascular system must be functional. Although patients with end-stage brain tumors are suitable candidates for Phase I trials, their relative infrequency places few primary brain tumors in Phase I studies.

Phase II

A drug becomes available for Phase II trials after prerequisite Phase I data have established toxicity of the drug and one or more appropriate schedules for its administration. The objective of a Phase II trial is to determine the antitumor activity (or inactivity) of a drug against one or more tumor types. As a result of Phase II trials, useful drugs become available for Phase III studies and for additional Phase II studies of drug combinations.

The author's present criteria for Phase II patient selection are:

(1) Patients must have a primary tumor of the neuraxis confirmed histologically. Patients with cerebral metastatic tumors, highly selected patients with intrinsic tumors of the dominant hemisphere, corpus callosum, thalamus, and brainstem may be accepted into the study without histologic confirmation if no alternative diagnosis is entertained. All patients must show a measurable tumor mass on a brain scintiphoto, radiographic contrast studies, or both, and most important, must manifest progressive neurologic deterioration (the rationale for this last criterion will be detailed in the discussion of patient evaluation below).

(2) Patients who have received radiation therapy can be accepted into Phase II trials if at least three months has passed since the end of therapy. It is assumed that after three months no further beneficial effects of radiation will occur, and that the patient has passed the period of transient neurologic deterioration occasionally observed six to twelve weeks after radiation therapy.[1]

(3) Prior chemotherapy does not preclude a patient's entry into a Phase II study. The only provision is that chemotherapy has been terminated at least eight weeks before the patient's acceptance; this ensures that delayed improvement and toxicity will be recognized. The use of corticosteroids and any form of anticonvulsant medication does not exclude a patient from a Phase II study.

(4) The patient, or the responsible family member, must give written consent to experimental treatment after hearing and understanding a full explanation of all factors involved (this is also required for Phase I and Phase III studies).

(5) Patients should have an estimated life expectancy of at least eight weeks. Many patients become worse shortly after starting chemotherapy and improvement beyond pretreatment status may require several weeks. Conversely, deaths occurring within eight weeks of treatment may not be due to the tumor's unresponsiveness. A responsive tumor swells to varying degrees before nonviable cells are lysed and absorbed, and within the brain significant reduction of bulk may require many days or even weeks. The key factors in selecting patients for Phase II trials are an evaluable mass and a progressively deteriorating clinical course.

Phase III

A Phase III trial is prospective, requires a control group or groups, and adheres to strict criteria for patient assignment in order to ensure significant data. A Phase III study compares the effects of chemotherapy, administered alone or in combination with other adjunctive therapy, with the effects of conventional ("best known") forms of therapy for a specific tumor type. Customarily, Phase III trials are carried out as the definitive initial treatment using a drug either alone or concurrently with other forms of therapy. Phase III trials differ in this respect from Phase II trials in which recurrent tumors have been treated unsuccessfully at an earlier time. A form of therapy whose effectiveness exceeds "best known" treatment in a Phase III trial becomes the best available therapy, and subsequent Phase III trials will use this form of therapy as the "best known" treatment for comparison with newer therapeutic approaches.

Study variables are reduced to a minimum by the following criteria for acceptance of patients into a Phase III study involving malignant gliomas:

(1) The diagnosis of primary malignant brain tumor must be confirmed histopathologically by craniotomy and subtotal removal of tumor. This criterion eliminates cases of metastatic and nonmalignant lesions and excludes astrocytomas of lower grade.

(2) The tumor must be supratentorial. Since the course of a malignant glioma in the posterior fossa may differ significantly from the course of a comparable tumor situated above the tentorium, patients with posterior fossa tumors are excluded from the study.

It is assumed that the growth rate of supratentorial tumors does not depend on their location. Although most neurosurgeons perform more extensive internal decompressions done in the nondominant hemisphere, patients are not stratified on this basis. However, the extent of internal decompression should be recorded for retrospective analysis.

(3) Patients must enter the study within a definite period after operation. The time limit is arbitrary but essential to assure comparability of patients.

(4) Corticosteroids can be used before, during, and after operation, but their use may be restricted once the patient enters the study. Scientific, moral, and practical considerations will establish future limitations for the use of corticosteroids in individual studies.

(5) Patients with a concomitant major medical, psychiatric, or other neurological illness must be excluded from the study. In such cases, drug activity may be altered, toxic effects amplified, and neurologic assessment drastically complicated.

(6) As in all other studies, valid consent for treatment must be obtained, and this includes informing the patient that the form of treatment, i.e. experimental versus "best known", will be determined from random selection.

Pregnancy

Although the situation arises rarely, the matter of accepting a patient with suspected or known pregnancy into a study deserves comment. Stutzman[2] has reviewed the sparse literature on this subject. On the basis of both animal and human data he concluded that drug treatment concurrent with or shortly after impregnation will precipitate destruction of the embryo. Drug treatment during the first trimester of gestation will cause either spontaneous abortion or a significant risk of fetal malformation. During the second and third trimesters, many drugs have caused no adverse effects in either animals or humans, and Brent has shown that hemotoxicity present in the mother at the time of birth may not be manifest in the infant.[3] Thus, administration of certain classes of drugs (i.e. antimetabolites, pyrimidine analogs) in the second and third trimesters would appear to be reasonably safe. However, some of the nitrosoureas have produced tumors in offspring of pregnant rats and rabbits injected during the latter half of gestation,[4] and conceivably they could do so in humans.

If chemotherapy is indicated during the first trimester, the fetus can be aborted with medical justification. If treatment with procarbazine or nitrosourea is started in any phase of pregnancy, abortion is probably indicated.

EVALUATION

Pretreatment Evaluation

Pretreatment studies establish a baseline for future assessment of the patient's neurologic condition, i.e. his response or lack of response to treatment. Preliminary studies also establish the functional state of organs that may be affected by drug toxicity. The tests described here are necessary in both Phase II and Phase III studies. In Phase I studies, less emphasis is placed on the neurologic tests, although serial clinical examinations are still required to evaluate possible neurotoxic side effects of any agent and especially if preclinical testing indicates neurotoxicity.

The fastest and most efficient way to obtain baseline studies is in the hospital, regardless of the patient's condition. Patients undergo: (1) general physical and detailed neurologic examinations, (2) complete blood count with platelet determination, (3) urinalysis, (4) determination of serum levels of BUN (blood urea nitrogen), creatinine, alkaline phosphatase, bilirubin, SGOT (serum glutamic oxaloacetic transaminase), LDH (lactic dehydrogenase), and postprandial blood sugar, (5) psychologic assessment in cases where this may be a sensitive index of neurologic change, (6) electroencephalography (EEG), (7) relevant contrast radiographic studies such as angiography, pneumoencephalography, or myelography unless current films of acceptable quality have been obtained prior to referral, (8) technetium pertechnetate brain scintiphoto, and when available, computerized axial tomography (CAT) scan for all intracranial tumors, and (9) cerebrospinal fluid collection for cytologic examination, if clinically judicious. Occasionally, when a drug is known to have unusual toxic side-effects, other specific baseline tests are needed, for example, with bleomycin therapy, chest X-rays and pulmonary function tests.

Reevaluation

Patients usually receive repeated courses of drug therapy at intervals of one to two months. In the majority of cases, neurologic deterioration (or improvement) occurs gradually and interim neurologic evaluation is not attempted. In practice, bone marrow toxicity (manifested by leukopenia, thrombocytopenia, and rarely, anemia) is the only side-effect for which routine serial interim testing has been necessary. This toxicity is the main dose-limiting factor for almost every drug now in use, and some degree of toxicity is seen in virtually every patient. With drugs such as methotrexate and cyclophosphamide, the nadir of peripheral blood counts occurs during the first two weeks after therapy; with BCNU and procarbazine, toxicity does not appear until the fourth to sixth week. Routinely, twice weekly complete blood counts with platelet determinations for all patients are obtained during the interval between treatments. These blood counts are performed in laboratories near the patient's home; the results are then forwarded to the hospital and flow sheets maintained for each patient. If the peripheral white blood count drops below 2000/mm³ and/or the platelet count below 35,000/mm³, daily determinations are ordered until values return to these levels.

With few exceptions, patients are admitted to the hospital for reassessment and retreatment, but when repeat radiographic studies are not required, when the treatment procedure itself does not require hospitalization, and when the patient is at least ambulatory with help, reevaluation and retreatment can be done on an outpatient basis.

Evaluation at the time of retreatment consists of: (1) general physical and neurologic examinations, (2) repetition of all blood chemistry tests obtained at the time of initial evaluation, (3) urinalysis, (4) technetium brain scintiphoto, and recently, CAT* scan, (5) CSF cytology and psychologic tests as indicated, and (6) EEG.

Prior to July, 1970, the author repeated angiographic studies on the majority of patients at the time of each admission for treatment. However, analysis of serial angiograms indicated a 40 percent positive correlation between the angiographic changes and the patient's clinical status,[5] whereas there was a 65 percent positive correlation between serial brain scintiphoto changes and clinical status in the same patients.[6] Subsequently we have discontinued angiography for serial evaluation and restricted its use to cases in which brain scintiphoto and clinical changes disagree and in patients for whom reoperation is under consideration.

Assessment of Response

The obvious and most important objective of the clinical and laboratory reassessment is an answer to the question: Has the patient's tumor regressed under treatment? In evaluating brain tumors there are three possible ways of answering this question.

The first is a method of the future. It will involve serial measurement of some biochemical or immunologic substance that is unique to the tumor, is present in cerebrospinal fluid and/or serum, and can be correlated quantitatively with viable tumor mass. Such substances currently under investigation are desmosterol (a cholesterol precursor)[7] aldolase-C,[8] and the polyamines

---

*Computerized Axial Tomography

putrescine, spermidine, and spermine,[9,10] all found in cerebro-spinal fluid. In the same way, it is hoped that neuroimmunologic studies will discover antibodies to tumor-specific antigens in the serum or CSF of brain tumor patients that can be correlated serially and quantitatively with the tumor mass.

These new, more direct methods of measurement are being sought because the current means for determining the tumor's response to treatment are indirect and imprecise. Presently employed methods are: (1) comparison of changes in the patient's neurologic status over serial treatment intervals, and (2) comparison of changes in serial brain scintiphotos, CAT scans, or serial EEG's done at the time of each readmission. Although there appears to be a high correlation between the EEG and responsivity to chemotherapy, the author has not used this as a major criterion of response.[11]

In evaluating neurologic improvement as a criterion of tumor regression, one should recognize that neurologic deficits, even those appearing immediately prior to treatment, may be irreversible. In such cases, the arrest of clinical deterioration, associated with a stable or improving brain scintiphoto, may be the only indication of response to therapy. The patient's condition must be deteriorating at the time of treatment in order to differentiate postsurgical neurologic impairment from dynamic deterioration secondary to tumor regrowth. Although one could argue that maintenance of status quo for a period of three to six months with neither clinical nor brain scintiphoto deterioration constitutes a response to therapy, the author has designated such cases probable responders rather than unequivocal responders.

It is now recognized that significant tumor cell kill may cause deterioration rather than improvement in neurologic function. In untreated glioblastomas one-third or more of the tumor mass (notably central areas) may be nonviable, and in these areas little if any phagocytic response is evident, even in necrotic areas that may be weeks old. Even if the chemotherapeutic agent kills a significant proportion of viable tumor cells, the disposal of dead cells by lysis and phagocytosis is so inefficient that total tumor mass remains grossly unchanged. In fact, the tumor-drug interaction may cause peritumoral edema, swelling of damaged tumor cells and expansion of extracellular space within the tumor with the net effect being a significant increase in mass effect.

Paradoxically, the most effective oncolytic agents may produce devastating and potentially fatal iatrogenic changes in neurologic function and intracranial pressure. This circumstance also affects the interpretation of serial brain scintiphotos as an index of tumor volume. Radionuclide images do not permit differentiation of viable and nonviable tumor from edema in adjacent and otherwise normal white matter. It is hoped that scintiphoto scans together with the CAT scan will allow such differentiation.

Corticosteroids

In Phase II studies, improvement due to the use of corticosteroids must be differentiated from improvement produced by oncolytic effectiveness of the agent under study. The variable amount of cerebral edema associated with both primary and metastatic neoplasms and the rapid, often dramatic clinical improvement observed after the systemic administration of corticosteroids are matters of record. These agents reduce cerebral edema already present and may inhibit its further formation for variable periods of time. Clinical improvement in patients receiving steroids has been credited to the reversal of physiologic dysfunction in edematous but otherwise intact brain and in some instances to an accompanying reduction of elevated intracranial pressure.

Suppose a patient with manifest symptoms from a recurrent glioblastoma is accepted into a Phase II study. Neurologic deterioration between the first and second courses is reversed by the administration of corticosteroids (either initiating or increasing the dose of maintenance therapy). At the time of readmission for the second course, any neurologic improvement over the initial status cannot be attributed to the oncolytic agent, and the patient cannot be labeled a responder.

Despite the difficulties posed by concurrent administration of corticosteroids, a high proportion of patients entering Phase II trials will require maintenance steroid therapy during the first few courses of chemotherapy, and for this reason, it is impractical to reject patients from a study because of steroid dependence. Rather, rigid criteria can be constructed for the interpretation of drug response in patients concurrently receiving steroids. The guidelines the author followed in Phase II studies are: (1) If a patient has been started on maintenance steroid therapy by the referring physician, during the initial evaluation the dosage is titrated to the minimum required to maintain a stable neurologic condition. The neurologic examination recorded after the patient has reached a stable state for seventy-two hours on a minimal maintenance steroid dose will be used as the patient's clinical baseline. (2) During the first and subsequent intervals following initial treatment, the author controls the dosage of steroids, usually after repeated consultation with the family. Seldom has he obtained significant neurologic improvement attributable to the chemotherapeutic agent within four weeks of the initial course of treatment. Consequently, he does not lower a maintenance dose of steroid during the first interval even if the patient's condition remains the same or improves. Many agents, the nitrosoureas in particular, have delayed oncolytic effects, and often because of unimpaired tumor growth in the first weeks following initial chemotherapy, he increases the steroid dose to maintain clinical stability. This circumstance usually arises in patients requiring maintenance steroids in the pretreatment period.

To interpret response to chemotherapy under these conditions, the authors adhere to the following rules: (1) If a patient continues the same dosage of corticosteroids for at least two consecutive treatment intervals, clinical and scintiphoto comparisons are valid in determining response (or lack of it); (2) If a patient's minimal maintenance steroid dosage was tapered and stopped over a treatment interval and his condition improved, or remained stable, he is designated a probable responder; and (3) Conversely, if steroids have been started or increased during treatment and the patient's condition remains the same or deteriorates, he is designated a nonresponder.

In a Phase III study, the use of corticosteroids presents a problem. Clearly, the beneficial effect of corticosteroids must be considered in evaluating if the end point is survival (see the section on "End Points").

To summarize: At present, it is believed that the comparison of serial changes in a patient's neurologic status provides the most reliable means of determining chemotherapeutic response in Phase II studies. Since the major criterion for acceptance in a Phase II trial is progressive neurological deterioration, any subsequent clinical improvement (unrelated to steroids) can be attributed to the chemotherapeutic agent. Currently, serial brain scintiphoto is the most accurate correlate to the clinical impression, although viewed retrospectively it gives misleading information in approximately 25 percent of cases.[12] Computerized axial tomography offers exciting promise as an objective means of defining the response of both tumor and adjacent brain to steroids, oncolytic agents, and other therapeutic modalities.

End Points

Occasionally during the course of therapy another form of treatment (e.g., reoperation, shunting) may be in the patient's best interest. If this alternative plan is adopted, violation of protocol will result in the patient's being dropped from the drug trial although the data obtained to that point can be considered in the final analysis.

For patients who respond to chemotherapy in Phase II trials, one could set a time limit beyond which a patient is considered "cured." At present the author's experience does not support a definitive conclusion, but with anaplastic gliomas one might suspect that a reasonable end point is two years of chemotherapy with no evidence of disease followed by an equal period of no treatment without evidence of regrowth.

The end point for Phase II studies is the time at which regrowth is identified either by clinical deterioration or by an enlarging brain scan abnormality. No useful information will be gained by knowing the period between regrowth and death. Once regrowth (recurrence) is documented, these patients should be placed on another protocol if their life expectancy is two months or longer. Only in this way is further prolongation of useful life possible and in no other way can information be obtained on drug cross-resistance.

On the other hand, in a Phase III trial, death has been the end point, since a "best known" treatment is being compared to an experimental therapy. As an end point, death provides a definitive and uncontested comparison of life expectancy in treated patients. Unfortunately, in the context of a Phase III study, there is no alternative point in time, although time from initial treatment to regrowth would be a much more reasonable end point. If, in current Phase III trials, first evidence of regrowth has a predictable relationship to death, the former can and should become the end point for future Phase III trials.

REFERENCES

1. Boldrey, E.B., and Sheline, G.: Delayed transitory clinical manifestations after radiation treatment of intracranial tumors. *Acta Radiol [Ther] (Stockh)*, 5:5, 1966.
2. Stutzman, L., and Sokal, J.E.: Use of anticancer drugs during pregnancy. In Hreshchyshyn, M.M. (Ed.): *Chemotherapy of Gynecologic Cancer*, vol. 11, no. 2 of *Clinical Obstetrics and Gynecology*. New York, Hoeber, 1968, pp. 416-427.
3. Brent R.L., Bolden, B.T., and Weiss, A.: The use of uterine vascular clamping in the pregnant rat to modify the embryotoxic effect of anticancer drugs. *Cancer Res, 28*:2001, 1968.
4. Druckrey, Hermann, Ivankovic, Stanislov, Preussmann, Rudolf, et al.: Selective induction of malignant tumors of the nervous system by resorptive carcinogens. In Kirsch, Wolff, Grossi Paoletti, Ernest, and Paoletti, Pietro (Eds.): *The Experimental Biology of Brain Tumors*. Springfield, Thomas, 1972, pp. 85-147.
5. Koo, A.H., Fewer, D., Wilson, C.B., and Newton, T.H.: Lack of correlation between clinical and angiographic findings in patients with brain tumors under BCNU chemotherapy. *J Neurosurg, 37*:9, 1972.
6. Handel, S.F., Powell, M.R., Wilson, C.B., and Enot, K.J.: Scintiphotographic evaluation of response of brain neoplasms to systemic chemotherapy. *J Nucl Med, 12*:292, 1971.
7. Weiss, J.F., Ransohoff, J., and Kayden, H.J.: Cerebrospinal fluid sterols in patients undergoing treatment for gliomas. *Neurology (Minneap), 22*:187, 1972.
8. Kumanishi, T., Ikuta, F., and Yamamoto, T.: Aldolase isozyme patterns of representative tumours in the human nervous system. *Acta Neuropathol (Berl), 16*:220, 1970.
9. Marton, L.J., Heby, O., and Wilson, C.B.: Increased polyamine concentrations in the cerebrospinal fluid of patients with brain tumors. *Inter J Cancer, 14*:731-735, 1974.
10. Marton, L.J., Heby, O., Wilson, C.B., and Lee, P.L.Y.: A method for the determination of polyamines in cerebrospinal fluid. *FEBS Lett, 46*:

305, 1974.

11. Spire, J., Renaudin, J., Calogero, J., and Wilson, C.B.: *The Electroencephalogram as an Indicator of Response to Brain Tumor Chemotherapy.* Presented at the Twenty-fifth Annual Meeting of the Neurosurgical Society of America, Pebble Beach, California, March 25, 1972.

12. Fewer, D., Wilson, C.B., Boldrey, E.B., et al.: The chemotherapy of brain tumors: clinical experience with carmustine (BCNU) and vincristine. *JAMA, 222:*549, 1972.

CHAPTER **SIX**

COORDINATING THE
CHEMOTHERAPY PROGRAM

K. JEAN ENOT

CHEMOTHERAPY IS A COMPLEX process involving diverse and highly experienced medical personnel whose efforts must be coordinated for efficient functioning of the program.

After referral to a treatment center, the brain tumor patient undergoes diagnostic studies, is assigned to an appropriate protocol, is instructed in all aspects of therapy and receives treatment over a period of time which will include readmissions for evaluation of therapy. In addition, the patient and his family will require guidance in hospital procedures and interpretation in various phases of the treatment. With the establishment of a chemotherapy program, it is vitally important to appoint a chemotherapy coordinator. In the early days of chemotherapy research, this position was usually filled by a physician. In the program of the authors of this book, the coordinator is a registered nurse. In some situations, a specially trained paramedical professional might also perform these duties.

Currently, about two hundred new brain tumor patients are admitted annually as candidates for treatment on the Chemotherapy Service of the Department of Neurological Surgery, University of California Hospitals, San Francisco (UCSF). The clinical staff of the service consists of the director, two principal investigators, the chemotherapy fellow, the chemotherapy coordinator, and the chemotherapy nurse. This coordinator is responsible for organizing and integrating the myriad details of each patient's treatment; she also assures the efficiency of treatment and the validity of research results by monitoring all aspects of therapy and confirming that protocols are strictly followed.

A chemotherapy coordinator spends more time with the patient

109

and his family than does any other member of the clinical staff. Because malignant brain tumors are fatal, the patient and his family will be seeking emotional support, comfort and reassurance. He or she also is the logical staff member to translate the technicalities of therapy into layman's language for the family and to allay anxieties arising from sometimes imposing complexities of modern medical technology. Conversely, the coordinator relays information gained in the course of counseling to the rest of the staff, thus insuring their awareness of the family's situation and feelings. Thus the coordinator assists the research team in maintaining the vital balance between the human concerns of the family and the scientific necessities of the chemotherapy program.

THE PATIENT AND THE RESEARCH PROGRAM

Referral

Currently, chemotherapy centers are few, and brain tumor patients are thus referred to them from a wide geographical area; many patients come from out of state. A referring physician's first contact with the chemotherapy program is often the coordinator, who can generally determine whether or not the patient is a suitable candidate for evaluation, based on the diagnosis, severity of neurological disability, and previous treatment, if any. As outlined in Chapter Five, only patients with a potential survivial time of eight weeks or longer can be considered for chemotherapy; a patient with a stable condition would make drug effect unevaluable and thus cannot be entered in Phase II trials. Patients who have undergone surgery more than three weeks previously cannot be considered for current Phase III studies.

The referring physician will be given complete information by letter on all details of the patient's hospitalization and treatment. Good communication is extremely important and requires that all consulting physicians involved in the case, e.g. ophthalmologists and neurologists, are fully informed and continually updated on the patient's course.

Admission

Once the patient is identified as a suitable candidate for the program, the coordinator must establish who is to be the responsible party. Each patient must have either a responsible family member or legal guardian to make necessary arrangements for care, give legal permission for participation in the program and make decisions regarding continuation or termination of therapy. If no such person is present, the patient is not accepted into the program.

The coordinator schedules the patient for admission to the hospital, stressing to him and his family that hospitalization at this point is only for evaluation and recommendation concerning treatment. Date of admission depends upon such factors as severity of symptoms, proximity of the patient's home to the chemotherapy center (such as UCSF), and time required for his family to make transportation arrangements. If his condition is deteriorating rapidly, the patient is usually admitted immediately for evaluation and initiation of treatment. Admission is often postponed for patients who have recently undergone irradiation to provide adequate time for the delayed effects of radiation therapy.

During its weekly rounds, the research team decides on diagnostic studies indicated (brain scan, EEG, pneumoencephalogram, arteriogram, psychological testing — if a pneumoencephalogram or arteriogram has been done recently, the study is seldom repeated), and the coordinator then schedules necessary studies with the appropriate hospital departments.

After admission for diagnostic studies, the patient's clinical status is evaluated daily by the principal investigator, the chemotherapy fellow, and the coordinator. This neurological grading establishes a baseline for judging therapeutic effectiveness and contributes to the planning of the overall program. Consultations are arranged for any concomitant medical problems which require attention.

Counseling

During this initial period, the coordinator initiates counseling with the patient and family. This service is a critical factor in assisting both to deal with the devastating effects of a terminal illness, particularly in the program's experimental context.

From the outset, the coordinator must establish a candid, but respectful relationship with patient and family. Communication may be impeded by the effects of the patient's disease, e.g. aphasia, euphoria, or confusion. In cases of dysphasia, the coordinator learns from the patient's family about his home and work background, his essential personality, and the present home situation. Then, speaking with the patient in private, he attempts to discuss matters with him on his own level, including a full description of the chemotherapy, what he will undergo and the expected effects. Observing the patient's reactions, the coordinator clarifies and expands the description as much as necessary. On this basis, the patient's willingness or unwillingness to participate in the project can usually be determined. If not, responsibility for the decision then rests with the family or legal guardian. Despite an apparent mental disability, the patient is fully informed of all decisions and treatment details throughout the study.

In the early interviews, the family's awareness of the illness is also assessed; this includes their comprehension of its terminal nature, their acceptance of the uncertainty of chemotherapeutic effect and areas that will require further counseling or clarification in future sessions..

Initially, the coordinator emphasizes that the cause of malignant brain tumors is unknown and that the disease is not inheritable, nor transmissable to others. The family is assured that no factors within their control contributed to the development of a tumor of this type, nor could earlier diagnosis and treatment have changed its inexorable course. A point that is stressed throughout the course of treatment is that the patient has and continues to receive optimal medical care.

During the initial visit, the family is also advised that chemotherapy is still considered an "extraordinary therapeutic measure" to maintain life, and that by rejecting it, they need not feel they have failed the patient in any sense. Should the patient or his family reject chemotherapy, the services remain available to assist them in any way possible and they are informed that they are naturally welcome to return for evaluation should they reconsider at a later time.

Patients and families alike benefit psychologically from an understanding of this particular program in relation to the overall field of brain tumor research. From this perspective, they comprehend more readily the value of their own participation in the program. In addition, the family may derive, in part, an emotionally supportive basis for reconciling their grief.

Counseling interviews also provide the coordinator with an opportunity to obtain information concerning the family's financial situation, so that she can help to arrange for state aid or other financing where necessary. She must also determine the emotional and physical climate in the home, directing attention to any special problems she perceives, or in some cases, advising psychiatric consultation. These problems, e.g., psychosocial pathology, excessive dependence of the patient's spouse, or potentially harmful effects on young children in the household are taken into consideration with other factors in determining if the patient can be cared for at home. Usually, the family is enthusiastic about keeping the patient at home as long as he is aware of where he is and they are able, with assistance, to meet his needs. The coordinator can begin at this time to assist the family in locating and utilizing community facilities and resources for assistance.

Protocol Assignment

Following evaluation and initial counseling, the chemotherapy team assigns the patient to an appropriate protocol. (Protocol requirements are described in Chapter Five.) If the tumor is metastatic or represents regrowth, the patient is automatically assigned to a Phase II study; the specific study to which he is assigned depends on several factors. If deteriorating rapidly, he may be treated according to a protocol on which response is expected within an early phase of treatment. Diagnosis, drug action and tumor characteristics are important factors, but other considerations, such as family situation and proximity of the patient's home to the chemotherapy center, are also taken into account. In extraordinary circumstances, such as extreme financial need coupled with distant residence, the coordinator can sometimes make special arrangements. For example, one child in the author's program receives therapy from a local physician who was formerly connected with the UCSF center, and the child reports to UCSF only once annually.

The family is familiarized with all details of the patient's specific protocol; this includes a detailed consent form and a written information sheet that stresses the protocol's experimental nature. (For sample forms, see Appendices.) These forms are explained verbally and rephrased or expanded until they are clearly understood. Written consent must be truly informed, an understanding that must be demonstrated by the patient and/or his family in their description, using their own words, of exactly what the treatment protocol involves.

If the patient is to be randomized to a protocol, this procedure as well as its alternatives, is detailed in both written and oral explanations.

Once the patient has been assigned to a specific study, the coordinator ensures that the treatment protocol is strictly followed.

Treatment

When treatment is initiated, the coordinator simultaneously begins instructing the family about the dosage, probable side-effects, and warning signs of serious toxicity of the medication the patient receives. Since most chemotherapy agents now in use cause nausea and vomiting three to four hours after administration, this side-effect is noted in the agreement for treatment which the patient and/or his family signs. Medications the author currently uses are administered either orally or by intravenous (I.V.) drip. (Dosage for all drugs is calculated per square meter of body surface area.) This simplicity of administration is very reassuring to the family, and young children can receive treatment in their own beds, with minimal discomfort.

Administration of oral medication is carefully timed according to its particular side-effects. Patients who are to receive medication causing nausea and vomiting usually are given a normal breakfast and lunch and receive their medication late in the afternoon. Consequently, adequate oral intake for the day is assured and supplementary I.V. fluids are avoided. Similarly, medications causing extreme drowsiness are given at bedtime.

Patients receiving a drug with an intermittent high dose schedule, e.g. once monthly administration, will be treated exclusively in the hospital. Those receiving medications in long-term daily doses start therapy in the hospital, then continue it at home. When the patient is discharged, the family is given only enough medication to complete one course of therapy, and at each subsequent hospitalization they are issued only enough additional medication to complete that particular course. Since corticosteroids are often a part of the patient's regimen, these medications must be explained to the family. Extra explanation may have to be given on dosage, since the family may be confused by the several sizes of tablets comprising the total dose. The family must be taught to read the labels of the medication packages. It is helpful to point out that there are alternate trade names for the same corticosteroid.

If the patient is to be cared for at home, the family is given instructions by the coordinator in seeing to his needs — administering medications, assuring an adequate oral intake, amount and kind of exercise and social stimulation allowable, amount of rest required, and so forth. She answers any questions the family may have on these subjects and allays their anxieties as much as possible. The coordinator also gives information on seizure precautions: She explains to the family the nature of seizures, emphasizes that seizures do not cause permanent brain damage, suggests that they time the seizures, tells them how to protect the patient, tries to help them accept the fact of seizures as a part of the illness, and helps them deal with their anxiety, for example, by telling them to remember that when the patient's color is at its worst and he looks the most frightening is when the seizure is just about to end.

Discharge Planning

The coordinator also oversees discharge planning. If the family does not have a regular family physician, they will need help in finding one. The patient's medical condition, plus any unusual family circumstances uncovered during counseling, will determine where he is to be sent. If the patient needs continued hospitalization, arrangements may have to be made with a hospital closer to his home community. If the patient is to be admitted to a convalescent hospital, the coordinator will assist the family in finding an appropriate facility, or if the patient is to live at home, the coordinator will help the family make whatever arrangements are necessary to facilitate home care. She determines what special equipment will be needed for home care and helps the family obtain it. The American Cancer Society frequently gives invaluable assistance in this regard. Arrangements can also be made to have a visiting nurse come regularly to the home to aid the family in caring for the patient. The coordinator must see that arrangements are made for the patient to have regular blood studies done in a laboratory near his home, and if other physicians are involved in the patient's care, he must monitor all treatment between visits to the medical center. Finally, the coordinator makes certain that transportation is arranged for returning the patient from the medical center to his home community.

On the day of discharge, the family is given the medication and an envelope of instructions. Written instructions for convalescent hospital personnel, family physician, or anyone else who is to be involved in the patient's care are also included.

In the interim periods between admissions to the medical center for reevaluation, the patient and his family are closely followed by the coordinator. If the patient lives nearby, he will come in for outpatient visits as needed with the coordinator or the chemotherapy fellow. If he lives farther away, his course will be followed by telephone. The coordinator and the chemotherapy fellow alternate on call at all times, so that the family can telephone at any time to discuss any new symptoms or problems that may arise and to receive continuing reassurance. They are encouraged to call even with small questions. Families on the whole are very considerate and seldom abuse this privilege. And as they begin to feel more secure, the number of calls decreases.

Reevaluation Admissions and Later Counseling

The patient will undergo subsequent admissions to the medical center for reevaluation and possible retreatment. At these times, the coordinator continues counseling. She determines whether the family has any new financial or other needs. She continues their education concerning the patient's routine medication, so that they may become increasingly intelligent participants in the therapy. The family's understanding of the medication should progress from knowing the number of each color of tablets that the patient receives daily to knowing the names of the drugs and the size in milligrams of the doses. Further counseling of the family also increases their comfort with the research program. At each visit, the coordinator reconfirms with the patient and his family their decision to continue participation in the program.

Along with education and practical assistance, the coordinator will also be giving continued emotional support to the family. An important part of this counseling is the removal of the family's guilt concerning the patient's illness. They must be reassured as often as necessary that whatever they have done for the patient is fine, that taking the patient to a physician earlier would not have appreciably changed the course of the illness, and that the patient has received and is receiving the best possible care from them.

Although the great majority of patients have communicative or cognitive problems, those who are able to comprehend and discuss the fact of their own death will need counseling as much as their families do. The patient who has grown to trust the coordinator will eventually broach the subject of his worries and fears, frequently blurting them out at unexpected times, e.g. on holidays or at a time when the coordinator is leaving for a trip. Thus the coordinator must take care never to give, verbally or nonverbally, a message of not being willing to listen, being acutely sensitive to signals from the patient when he may need to talk; if she suspects the patient is ready to discuss his feelings, she should make certain that she is readily available. Patients frequently are concerned about and want to discuss both practical and personal matters: Will the family be financially secure? Who will care for young children? Will the spouse remarry? The patient will also want to share and discuss his emotions concerning his own death.

Children in Treatment

Approximately 5 percent of the patients in our studies have been children. They are usually admitted with either brain stem gliomas, treated either initially or as regrowth, or with recurrent medulloblastomas.

Even very young children are able to cooperate with treatment, and by about age five they are able to discuss their illness and understand simple explanations, although they have no concept of death before approximately age nine. The coordinator explains as much about the illness and treatment to the child as he can in the child's own terms. It is best to be matter-of-fact and direct with children and teenagers, who often respond better to this approach than do adults. Children are extremely resilient, and tend to adjust more easily than adults to disability. Too much solicitude from an overprotective mother, especially when a child is doing well under treatment and is eager to be active, may also have to be dealt with by the coordinator. Teenagers may have special problems with plans for the future, and the coordinator should cover these concerns in counseling. She must help the teenager to be realistic about his disabilities and shape his vocational or other plans accordingly.

Parents of children with brain tumors tend to have more emotional difficulties than families with sick adult members. They are especially likely to have more guilt and feel that something they have done in some way caused the child to have the tumor. The death of a child is more devastating to a family structure and more likely to create family pathology than is the death of an adult member; thus expert counseling from the coordinator becomes even more important in these situations. Chemotherapy of a child with a painful terminal disease is emotionally exhausting to the whole clinical staff.

Termination of Therapy

The coordinator must be sensitive to any hints the family may give concerning how they wish to handle the patient's impending death. If chemotherapy is continued past the time when it is having any effect on the patient's disease, it can place an added emotional burden on the family. They may have continued to care for the patient at home as long as they can endure, but it may be difficult for them to express such feelings directly. The coordinator can sometimes help the family to reach a decision by voicing the weariness and discouragement she may sense they feel. The coordinator must also communicate the family's feelings to the rest of the clinical staff, suggesting termination to the physicians as well as the family. If the family has difficulty in accepting the progressive decline of the patient, they may feel comforted by having the responsibility for the decision to terminate therapy taken by the physician. Families are usually relieved by a suggestion that therapy be stopped, as this leaves them emotionally free to enter the grieving processs without further false hopes that something still might be done for the patient. The coordinator assures them that even after termination of therapy they and the patient will receive whatever medical and emotional support they need. Should the family adamantly insist on continuation of chemotherapy and unusual means of life support until the patient's death, therapy is prolonged past the time when it has ceased to demonstrate any effectiveness.

Death

The great majority of patients in the author's program survive only a matter of months; only four have been followed for as long as four years. When the patient dies, the coordinator assists the family with the decision concerning the autopsy and other necessary arrangements. She tries to assure that the details of all final arrangements are carried out as planned, including follow-up to be sure the autopsy has been performed promptly.

Frequently, the family will undergo a period, immediately after the patient's death, of euphoria and relief. Subsequently, they will feel guilty for having such reactions. The coordinator should support and encourage the family during this period, assuring them that these feelings are entirely normal. She helps the family deal with their grief, encouraging them to release their emotions. This support is continued until the family is over the acute phase of the reaction to the patient's illness and death and has resumed a more or less normal life. Even after this, the coordinator may send a Christmas card or make an occasional friendly phone call, just to see how the family is doing and to relay the message, "We care."

Family Support as a Program Goal

Of course, the ultimate goal of any cancer chemotherapy program is cure of the patient. Given the current state of brain tumor therapy, however, this factor is not within the control of the coordinator or other staff members of the program. What is within their control is the more immediate goal of assuring the family of the continuing help and support they need and of the research of which they have been a part. If the family does feel cared for and supported, the program has been beneficial, at least from the coordinator's point of view.

Notes of gratitude received by this chemotherapy coordinator from patients' families have been strikingly uniform in their expression of the feeling that the brain tumor victim was treated as a person, not just another hospital patient, and that the coordinator and the chemotherapy team have been more like personal friends than professional helpers to the patient and his family. This quality should be actively sought in a chemotherapy program of this kind.

STATISTICS

Statistical data for later analysis in the research are collected by the coordinator through records kept on each patient: type and dosage of medication, response or lack of response, length and degree of response, toxicity, complications, and so on. Files are also kept for each patient containing hospital admissions and discharge summaries, laboratory reports, and correspondence with referring physician and consultants. For the many patients receiving chemotherapeutic agents which affect the bone marrow, the coordinator receives the laboratory reports by phone or mail and enters the weekly blood counts on a flow sheet. When counts approach a dangerous level, the coordinator may initiate daily blood counts to maintain a closer watch on the patient's condition or, if necessary, admit the patient to the hospital. Doses of concomitant medications, especially corticosteroids, must also be carefully recorded for consideration when effectiveness of the trial agent is being assessed. Accurate recording of all details concerning each patient's treatment course is of great importance for assessment of drug effectiveness and attainment of statistical significance in the research.

In addition to individual record keeping, the coordinator maintains running statistics on each study as a whole. These statistics can be consulted at any time to determine how many patients have participated in a particular study to that point and where the study stands. If an undesirable pattern seems to be emerging in the statitics, the coordinator calls this to the attention of the principal investigator.

Personnel in other hospital departments involved in the care of chemotherapy patients — nursing, physical therapy, nuclear medicine, neuroradiology — can be of greater assistance if they have an improved understanding of chemotherapy. At UCSF, the coordinator and the chemotherapy fellow have been leading informal seminars on the nature of chemotherapy and the goals of the program.

THE NURSE AS CHEMOTHERAPY COORDINATOR

The registered nurse who becomes a coordinator in a chemotherapy research program has the unique opportunity of performing a greatly expanded nursing role. The coordinator must be able to utilize a range of nursing knowledge and experience, and humanitarian ideals, in accomplishing more effective delivery of health care to the patient with a malignant brain tumor. She must be highly skilled not only in medical knowledge but in delicate interpersonal relationships, and be able to act in a strongly supportive manner. An excellent psychologist, skilled at picking up unspoken cues to peoples' feelings, and at helping them to feel comfortable enough to express their feelings freely, the coordinator must understand the mechanisms of guilt and grief and must know how to help people express repressed feelings and work through the many emotional stresses involved in facing the serious illness and death of a close family member. The coordinator must also be an educator, a social worker, and a communications expert.

The position of chemotherapy coordinator develops the nurse as a person. Since she is dealing exclusively with dying patients, and almost exclusively with short-term survivors, she must be able to talk about death, to think about death, and to develop her own personal philosophy about death. The position is emotionally exhausting and refreshing at the same time; such work can restore one's faith in humanity by giving the opportunity to view at close range the grace and courage with which dying persons and their families deal with an intolerable situation. Thus, while the coordinator is helping the family in dealing with their problems, she herself is learning and growing.

CHAPTER SEVEN

SPECIFIC AGENTS IN
BRAIN TUMOR CHEMOTHERAPY

DEREK FEWER

THIS CHAPTER DISCUSSES the agents employed in clinical chemotherapy of brain tumors — those used at the time this book was prepared, those that have been used in the past, and some drugs that may hold promise for future single and combination use.

Few clinical (Phase II) studies have shown an effect (or lack of effect) against brain tumors, and the literature contains only one completed study in which a drug was used as a form of primary, adjunctive therapy (Phase III). Many Phase II studies either have failed to stratify patients within the study according to the factors discussed in Chapter Five or have lacked sufficient numbers of patients. These studies have provided basic data on the various routes of administration, their advantages and complications. For each agent described, information on its development, mode and site of action determined by *in vitro* and/or *in vivo* testing, toxicity in humans, scheduling, and clinical results will be given where pertinent. The data are derived from the author's own experience and that of others reported in the literature.

AGENTS IN RECENT USE

BCNU

This agent, one of a number of nitrosourea derivatives synthesized at the Southern Research Institute in the early 1960's, has set the standard for *in vitro, in vivo,* and clinical testing against brain tumors. It is illustrative to trace the course of this drug from its development to the present time.

In 1960, Greene, et al. reported a significant antitumor effect of 1-methyl-3-nitro-1-nitrosourguanidine against intraperitoneal

L1210 leukemia in mice.[1] Many derivatives of this drug were then synthesized, one class of which was the nitrosoureas. The first drug of this class to be tested was methyl nitrosourea (MNU), and it was found effective in prolonging the lives of mice with intra-cerebrally inoculated L1210. An MNU derivative, BCNU (1,3-bis(2-chloroethyl)-1-nitrosourea), was found to be a superior drug against this same tumor system.[2]

At about the same time, Rall and Zubrod described the ideal characteristics for any compound that must cross the blood-brain barrier by diffusion: a high degree of lipid solubility, a low degree of ionization at physiologic pH and a low degree of plasma protein binding.[3] All of the nitrosourea derivatives, including BCNU, that were found active against intracerebral tumors have these characteristics.[2] In fact, BCNU reached high concentrations in normal mouse brain tissue after systemic administration[4]; water-soluble agents cannot do this. In dogs, BCNU was found to have a rapid half-life of about twenty minutes in plasma, reaching high concentrations in the CSF during the initial period after I.V. administration, but disappearing rapidly so that none could be found after two hours.[5]

Studies into its mechanism of action have shown that BCNU inhibits reactions necessary for purine biosynthesis and thus is, in effect, a DNA inhibitor.[6] It is believed to interfere with DNA function in the manner of alkylating agents.[7] Bruce tested BCNU in his AKR lymphoma system (see Chapter One), and found that the dose-survival plot is characteristic for a cycle-specific drug, thus making it a preferred agent for the initial chemotherapeutic treatment of a large tumor with a small growth fraction.[8] Wilkoff emphasized that cultured L1210 cells in a nonproliferative condition are also sensitive to BCNU.[4] It has not yet been proven whether this same effect occurs *in vivo*. Shapiro, et al. demonstrated a significant antitumor effect against three different intracerebrally implanted carcinogen-induced brain tumors in mice.[9] In the author's laboratory, BCNU proved effective against both carcinogen-induced glioma and human glioblastoma in cell culture as well as against rat glioma *in vivo*. Preliminary studies in man using ^{14}C labeled BCNU showed that the drug or its radioactive breakdown products rapidly entered the CSF and drug levels persisted there for nine hours.[10]

As early as 1963, BCNU was shown to be effective in clinical use against meningeal acute lymphocytic leukemia[11]; this observation with the above experimental findings made it a logical choice for use against intracerebral tumors. To date, two independent Phase II studies have been reported, and a cooperative Phase III study is nearing completion. In the Phase II studies response rates of 53 percent (16/30)[12] and 66 percent (6/9)[13] were observed for patients with malignant gliomas treated on nearly identical schedules. A significant number of positive responses was also seen in patients with brainstem gliomas and ependymomas although the number of such tumors was small. The majority of patients in both series had received radiation therapy as part of their initial treatment, but in all cases it had been completed at least one month prior to the initiation of chemotherapy. The concomitant use of systemic corticosteroids was also taken into consideration in the interpretation of response. The duration of response in this series is indicated in Table 7-I.

The dose-limiting toxicity of BCNU is a delayed depression of leukocytes and platelets; both Phase II studies illustrated the dose dependency of this toxicity. Using intensive intermittent therapy (100 to 125 mg/m^2 q.d., *quaque die*, x 3), Walker reported that platelet transfusion was necessary in fourteen of thirty-one courses of treatment (45%). In the author's own series, using starting dosages of 80-100 mg/m^2 every day for three days, transfusions for either serious thrombocytopenia or leukopenia were necessary in only eighteen of 169 courses (11%).

The depression of the platelets and leukocytes begins three to five weeks after treatment, with the platelets reaching a nadir about a week before leukocytes. This curious late onset of marrow depression has never been adequately explained. DeVita, et al.[10] have demonstrated that the prolonged plasma and tissue retention of ^{14}C-labeled breakdown products of BCNU is perhaps partly due to enterohepatic recirculation; it seems unlikely that this is the mechanism accounting for delayed toxicity. In most instances, counts return to normal six to eight weeks after treatment, at which time another course can be administered. In the author's experience, the hematoxicity of BCNU is cumulative.[12]

TABLE 7-I

LENGTH OF RESPONSE
AFTER INITIAL CHEMOTHERAPY WITH BCNU*

Length of Response in Months	Number of Patients Responding per Tumor Type					
	Glioblastoma	Astrocytoma	Ependymoma	Brain Stem Glioma	Melanoma	*Medullo-blastoma*
1	3	--	--	--	--	--
2	2	1	--	--	1	--
3	4	--	--	--	--	--
4	1	2	--	--	--	--
5	--	--	--	--	--	1
6	2	1	1	--	--	--
7	3	--	--	1	--	--
8	--	(1)	--	--	--	--
9	--	--	--	--	--	--
10	--	--	--	--	--	--
11	--	--	--	--	--	--
12	1	(2)	--	--	--	--
13	--	--	(1)	--	--	--
14	--	--	(1)	--	--	--

*Numbers in brackets indicate number of patients still under treatment at the cutoff point of this review in 1971.

To prevent an unacceptable degree of toxicity, he was forced to lower the total dosage of each course by 15 to 30 mg. Only twelve patients received the initial dose for two successive courses. This reduction of dosage is a possible cause of tumor regrowth in patients responding initially to BCNU.

Many patients experience nausea and vomiting shortly after

each dose of BCNU, but this has not compromised therapy. The author also observed elevation of serum SGOT, LDH, or alkaline phosphatase, but usually to no more than two to three times normal values. This occurred in the majority of patients but was not cumulative and was never associated with any clinical symptoms. Nevertheless, administration of BCNU to a patient with an already diseased liver should be done with caution since at high doses cirrhosis has been produced in dogs.[10]

In the BTSG Phase III study of BCNU now nearing completion, patients with malignant astrocytomas were randomized within three weeks of initial operation among protocols of BCNU alone, BCNU and radiation, radiation alone, and no further treatment. The end point was death, and length of survival was the dependent variable. The use of corticosteroids was limited, this factor an additional variable.

The preliminary results of this study have been reported by Walker and Gehan.[14] With 180 evaluable patients, the median survival according to group was: no treament, seventeen weeks; BCNU alone, twenty-eight weeks; irradiation alone, thirty-seven weeks; BCNU and irradiation, forty-one weeks. The rather poor results shown in this study for BCNU alone contrast with the good results obtained in the Phase II tests of BCNU. The fact that virtually all of the patients in the Phase II tests had already received a course of irradiation may be an important factor. The results of the Phase III study should stimulate basic research aimed at elucidating the mechanisms of the additive or synergistic effect of the nitrosoureas and irradiation.

BCNU represents the first chemotherapeutic agent effective in increasing the lifespan of patients with recurrent malignant brain tumors. In addition, it has not been uncommon in the author's experience to observe complete reversal of such findings as dysphasia, stupor, and hemiparesis in many patients who, when entered on the study, had a severe neurological deficit.

The encouraging results obtained with BCNU can serve as a baseline for determining effectiveness when reviewing clinical studies of other promising new drugs as they become available.

CCNU

CCNU (1-(2-chloroethyl)-3-cyclohexyl-1-nitrosourea) is another analog derivative of MNU. It is even more lipid soluble than BCNU[15] and has the advantage of oral administration.

Distribution studies in the mouse with ^{14}C-labeled CCNU have shown that the label readily enters and concentrates in normal brain as well as brain tumor tissue and that a plasma/brain ratio steady state is reached soon after administration.[16] When ^{14}C-labeled CCNU was administered to dogs as a single I.V. injection, radioactive levels in the CSF were two to three times greater than in plasma during the six-hour interval. As with BCNU, biotransformation of the parent CCNU occurs within minutes, and the majority of the radioactive byproducts are excreted by the kidneys within the hour.

CCNU was chosen for clinical trials because of its evident life-prolonging effect when used against intracerebral murine ependymoblastoma[16] and intracerebral L1210 leukemia.[10] Recently, Swenberg showed increased survival times in the CCNU treatment of rats with primary MNU-induced brain tumors.[17] This is perhaps the ultimate *in vivo* model and it should be used to screen other potentially useful agents. In a Phase I study, marked neurologic improvement occurred in three of three patients with malignant astrocytomas.[15]

On the basis of this background data, CCNU has undergone Phase II testing and two studies have been reported.[18,19,20] In a preliminary report, Walker [18] showed a 28 percent response rate after the first course, using 130 to 150 mg/m² in a single oral dose. Rosenblum updated this same series, reporting that the response rate was close to 40 percent (malignant astrocytoma and other brain tumors).[20] In the author's own series,[19] he reported a response rate of 33 percent in fifteen patients with malignant astrocytoma who had not had prior chemotherapy; the duration of response ranged from one to seven months. In addition, there were two responses out of five patients with metastatic disease (one carcinoma of the lung and one adenocarcinoma of unknown origin). In another group of eight patients (including four with malignant astrocytomas), who had previously been treated with BCNU and had either shown no response or had regressed, no response was observed. Although this latter group is small, this author feels certain that there exists a cross-resistance between these two similar drugs. An interesting improvement of neurologic signs in patients who showed no evidence of tumor progression (a group not usually considered for chemotherapy protocols) has also been reported.[20]

The recommended dose and schedule of this agent is 120 mg/m² given orally and repeated when hematologic values return to normal (in six to eight weeks). The dose-limiting toxicity is delayed bone marrow depression almost identical with that of BCNU, but with the dose and schedule used, no patient who had not had prior chemotherapy required transfusions.

One important point with regard to the hematoxicity of this drug is that in only one of seven patients who received three or more courses of CCNU was there observed a pattern of toxicity indicating a cumulative effect, and this was mild. Rosenblum, et al. showed lower nadir values for platelets after the fourth and fifth courses in a small number of patients, but their values were still within safe limits.[20] As a result, no patient received less than 85 percent of the initial dose. This is in sharp contrast to the author's experience with BCNU, where the cumulative toxicity was prominent in all but one case receiving more than two courses.

In summary then, CCNU is an effective agent against brain tumors and is comparable to BCNU.

Mithramycin

Mithramycin has been subjected to a number of Phase II studies and, on the basis of these studies, it was used in the first cooperative Phase III study undertaken by the Brain Tumor Study Group. It is an antibiotic, isolated from a strain of Streptomyces. Studies indicate that its primary mode of action is the blocking of RNA synthesis,[21] although it affects DNA and protein synthesis to some degree.[22] Mithramycin is not lipid soluble[23] but has been detected in CSF and tumor cyst fluid[24] after administration of the tritiated drug.

When it showed a positive, but not marked, antitumor effect in a number of animal systems, mithramycin was subjected to clinical trial. It aroused the interest of brain tumor chemotherapists because: (1) Central nervous system toxicity, reflected by transient drowsiness, restlessness, etc., was one of its prevalent toxic side-effects[25]; and (2) In one large Phase II study in which many different tumor types were included, a significant number of responses (eight of twenty) were noted in patients with metastatic brain tumors.[26,27]

Two Phase II studies aimed specifically at brain tumors have now been reported. Ransohoff, et al. reported clinical improvement in eight of fourteen patients harboring recurrent malignant gliomas, although for the most part the duration of improvement was brief.[24] Kennedy, et al. reported responses in four of nine patients treated with mithramycin for inoperable or recurrent malignant brain tumors; the responses lasted up to five months.[28] The dosage (25 to 50 mcg per kg/day IV x 1 day, every four weeks) used by them was far less than the dosage now considered optimal (25 to 30 mcg per kg/day x 8 to 10 days).[23] Laboratory studies indicated that mithramycin produced modest (30 to 40%) inhibition of growth in subcutaneously implanted Zimmerman ependymoblastoma in mice,[29] and that unique cytotoxic nuclear changes occurred in mithramycin-treated cultures of a variety of neural tumors, including many malignant gliomas.[30]

On the basis of laboratory and clinical observations, the BTSG designed a Phase III study of mithramycin. The findings were first reported in 1969.[31] In a reasonably well-controlled prospective study, there were ninety-six evaluable patients with either glioblastoma multiforme or malignant glioma. Patients began treatment within six weeks of their initial decompressive craniotomy; some received concomitant radiation therapy. The treated group had an average survival of 103 days from operation and the control group 117 days. One possible and likely reason for the poor result is the dosage used (25 mcg/kg/day x 21 days, repeated twice at six-week intervals) which was far in excess of that now recommended.

In a more recent experiment Shapiro, et al.[9] demonstrated that, in mice bearing intracerebral (as opposed to subcutaneous) implants of the Zimmerman ependymoblastoma, I.P. mithramycin caused an insignificant increase in survival. This experiment supports the author's view that the best *in vivo* drug screen for brain tumors is an intracerebral tumor model in which the agent acts in the same environment that it encounters in the clinical situation.

Methotrexate

Methotrexate, one of the first drugs to be employed in clinical chemotherapy, has been in continuous use for over twenty years. Effective either alone or in combination against many human tumors, it has without doubt been the subject of a larger volume of basic research than any other chemotherapeutic agent. Its known effectiveness against meningeal lymphocytic leukemia after I.T. administration[32] raised the hope that similar results could be achieved in primary brain tumors.

Methotrexate is a folic acid antagonist. In normally functioning cells, folic acid is reduced by a two-step reaction to tetrahydrofolic acid; both of these steps are believed dependent upon the enzyme dihydrofolic acid reductase. Derivatives of tetrahydrofolic acid act as important coenzymes which function as carbon carriers for many synthetic reactions, including: (1) the synthesis of thymidine acid (d TMP), a necessary step in DNA synthesis, and (2) purine synthesis, a necessary step for both DNA and RNA synthesis. Methotrexate acts by binding to the enzyme dihydrofolic acid reductase, thus effectively blocking both of the above reactions. It is thus a phase-specific drug as classed by Bruce, et al. (see Chapter One).[8]

Little work has been done with methotrexate in animal brain tumor models. Levin, et al.[33] showed that ^{3}H-methotrexate, administered I.P., enters the extracellular space and a 1 percent intracellular space in the murine intracerebral ependymoblastoma. Tator demonstrated with radioautography the uptake of tritiated methotrexate by tumor cells in an intracerebrally implanted murine ependymoblastoma.[34] Using a schedule of I.P. administration four times a day for four days, Shapiro was unable to increase the overall survival rate of mice bearing glioma 26, glioma 261 or ependymoblastoma A, although there were some long-term survivors.[9]. Thus, although methotrexate will cross the blood-tumor barrier in this tumor system, it cannot achieve an adequate concentration for the period of exposure required to be effective. Animal experiments utilizing I.T. (intrathecal) methotrexate present technical difficulties. The author performed one study in which rats bearing a transplanted mammary sarcoma and a cultured human oligodendroglioma had an increased average survival time after both I.P. and I.T. methotrexate but animals survived significantly longer after the I.T. therapy. The dosage used was 0.5 mcg/mg given two or three times at two day intervals starting on day four after implantation.

Methotrexate does not undergo metabolic alteration *in vivo*. After a single I.V. injection, maximum serum levels are achieved for one to two hours followed by a gradual decline to undetectable levels at twenty-four hours.[35] Ninety percent of a single I.V. dose of labeled methotrexate is excreted by the kidneys within twenty-four hours. After continuous oral or I.V. administration for a twenty-four hour period or longer, the drug can be detected in plasma for up to four days after the cessation of therapy.[35] In this same study, representative samples of tissue from many organs were retained at autopsy after labeled methotrexate had been given prior to death. Brain tissue contained the lowest amount of activity. This finding is in keeping with the physical characteristics of methotrexate, since it is not lipid soluble and binds to protein. If a constant systemic infusion is carried out in dogs so that plasma and CSF levels can equilibrate, the CSF/plasma ratio is .004. Tator[34] showed that tritiated methotrexate was taken up by the cells of the intracerebrally implanted rat ependymoblastoma, but the labeled drug was concentrated in the central areas of the tumors rather than in the periphery where most of the active growth occurs. Methotrexate is also actively excreted from the CSF by the cells of the choroid plexus.[36] The preceding observations indicate that systemic administration of low doses of methotrexate has little, if any, role in brain tumor chemotherapy.

However, methotrexate can be safely administered I.T.[32,37] and high CSF concentrations persisting at therapeutic levels for up to forty-eight hours have been achieved after a single injection in dogs.[37] After I.T. administration in dogs, methotrexate rapidly escapes into the systemic circulation, where it can cause toxic side-effects. The dose-limiting toxicity of methotrexate is bone marrow depression, evidenced by a reduction in the peripheral platelet and white blood cell counts. In contrast to the delayed appearance of this phenomenon with the nitrosoureas, the onset after methotrexate administration is usually within the first week for both elements, and it may take two to three weeks before recovery occurs, with leukocytes usually recovering first.[38]

The other major form of toxicity is gastrointestinal. Buccal mucosal ulceration is the initial manifestation, and unless therapy is stopped, potentially fatal hemorrhagic diarrhea will follow. Usually methotrexate can be restarted after one week's rest if stopped at the first sign of buccal ulceration. Other milder forms of toxicity are usually benign, e.g. alopecia, rash.

Up to 16 mg/kg of methotrexate can be safely administered systemically, but the availability of an antidote permits the safe use of much larger doses. The antidote is N5 formyl tetrahydro-folic acid (citrovorum factor, leucovorin), which *in vivo* is metab-olized to or is effective as tetrahydrofolic acid. It bypasses the block created by methotrexate, competes with methotrexate for uptake into cells and can displace intracellular methotrex-ate.[39]

A conversion product of leucovorin, 5-methyltetrahydrofolate, crosses the blood-brain barrier[40] and may neutralize some of the antitumor effects of methotrexate.[41] Consequently, much of the therapeutic advantage would be lost by the simultaneous admin-istration of leucovorin and methotrexate. Goldin has demon-strated that the delayed administration of leucovorin achieves a higher therapeutic index than the simultaneous administration of leucovorin and methotrexate.[42] This delay is possible because significant bone toxicity does not occur during the "unprotected" period (twenty-four to forty-eight hours), as explained by the work of Bruce.[8] Under conditions of normal bone marrow kin-etics, only a small fraction of the stem cells are in the proliferative pool, and even after a twenty-four hour exposure to methotrexate there will still be a substantial number of unaffected cells which subsequently can move out of the nonproliferative pool, enter the cell cycle, and repopulate the bone marrow. Precursor cells will reach maturity under the protection of leucovorin.

Dosage and scheduling within the limts of toxicity are critical because of acquired resistance to methotrexate. One proposed mechanism for resistance is that some tumor cells either possess or, under the influence of sublethal concentrations of methotrexate, develop the ability to produce excess dihydrofolic acid reductase and thus competitively neutralize the oncolytic effects of the drug.[43] Because levels of 5 x 10⁻⁶M are required to achieve a 95 percent inhibition of DNA synthesis,[44] in clinical use it is desirable to obtain the highest possible concentration of drug.

Based on these data, the concept of methotrexate-leucovorin rescue was described and tested clinically in patients with head and neck cancer.[39,45] It proved to be as effective as other intermittent therapy regimes but without increased acute or cumulative toxicity after many doses.

The author adapted this technique for I.T. use and accumulated Phase I data on eight patients. The method involved a twenty-four to forty-eight hour infusion of methotrexate at doses ranging from 80 to 240 mg/m² via the lumbar subarachnoid or intraven-tricular (via an Ommaya reservoir) routes. At the end of this period, leucovorin was administered (P.O., *per os*, or I.M.) at a dosage of 75 mg and followed by 15 mg every six hours for periods of thirty-six to one hundred thirty-two hours. The author administered up to 180 mg/m² over a forty-eight hour period with a rescue length of one and one-half to five days without any observable hematoxicity. In one patient with a recurrent ependymoma of the fourth ventricle he observed neurological improvement two weeks after a second course. Data would tend to confirm the lack of cumulative hematoxicity previously reported.[39] The Phase I study was abandoned without attempting to increase the dose and shorten the period of rescue.

Ojima and Sullivan[46] compared CSF and brain tissue levels of tritiated methotrexate after either single or continuous administration by I.V., I.A., or I.T. routes. Detectable levels were present in the CSF by all routes but were much higher by the I.T. route. A continuous I.T. infusion of only 5 mg/24 hours for seven days resulted in CSF levels one-half of the theoretically optimal concentration.[44] After continuous I.T. infusion, levels in the CSF declined slowly, with detectable drug still present two to three weeks after infusion. How long effective oncolytic concentrations persist is unclear. This is an important observation since it indicates the necessity of administering leucovorin for periods longer than the thirty-six hours known to be adequate after systemic administration of methotrexate.

In animals, I.T. methotrexate can cause seizures,[37] and the same has been observed in humans. Potentially more serious neurotoxicity in the form of subacute necrotizing encephalopathy, ascending myelitis, and aseptic meningitis has recently been reported and seems directly related to high concentrations of methotrexate in the cerebrospinal fluid.[47, 48, 49] Although these are isolated case reports, neurotoxicity may be more prevalent than is presently believed and may, in fact, be misinterpreted as relapse of leukemic meningitis or continued growth of solid tumors.

In most clinical studies the I.T. route has been used. However, partial short-term objective responses were reported following intracarotid infusions of methotrexate in seven of nine patients for periods up to two weeks; citrovorum factor was administered concomitantly.[50] Unfortunately, intracarotid infusion is a cumbersome method of delivery, with inherent risks. Sayers reported the results of treating forty-four children with one to six courses of I.T. methotrexate (using a dosage schedule of 0.25 mg/kg q.d. x 5 to 7 days).[51] He reported reversal of neurologic deficits as evidence of response occurring in 44 percent of the patients. Rubin, et al. using CSF perfusion techniques, reported seven patients with gliomas, five of whom improved symptomatically, two of these for a three month period.[52] Weiss and Raskind intermittently injected methotrexate directly into the tumor bed via an Ommaya device implanted at the time of surgery.[53] A dose of 0.25 mg/kg was barbotaged into the operative site every fifty-one days. The number of infusions was not indicated and no long-term followup was provided on the nine patients treated. At this dosage they observed no significant systemic toxicity.

In an early study of I.T. methotrexate before leucovorin rescue was initiated, responses of some medulloblastomas were dramatic and appear significant despite the small number of patients.[54, 55] Dramatic responses occurred in a reticulum cell sarcoma of the corpus callosum, a recurrent fourth ventricular ependymoma, and a recurrent medulloblastoma in the earlier series[54] and in two more patients with medulloblastomas in the later series.[55] There was a brief but clear response in one patient with a glioblastoma of the brain stem. Treatment in some cases was continued for periods up to two years. The favorable results of several clinical studies justifies the further use of this agent.

Methotrexate, being a phase-specific agent, is not an optimal drug for a large solid tumor with a small growth fraction. Its theoretical usefulness is either in combination with a cyclenonspecific agent which is used first to reduce the bulk of the tumor, and to move a larger percentage of tumor cells into the proliferative pool, or as surgical adjunctive therapy in a Phase III study.

Other antifolates have been synthesized and some have been found to cross the blood-brain barrier. NSC 139105, a triazine antifolate synthesized by the late B.R. Baker, has been evaluated in Walker 256 carcinosarcoma and L1210; it was found effective against the former but not the latter tumor.[56] In dogs, CSF drug level was 10 to 20 percent that of the level in plasma after I.V. administration.[56] However, in studies in the author's laboratories NSC 139105 did not cross the blood-brain barrier of mice or rats with any rapidity, nor was it effective in either the intracerebral rat gliosarcoma or murine glioma 26 tumor models.[57] Other agents with more promise are pyrimethamine and 2,4-diamino-5-(3′, 4′-dichlorophenyl)-6-methylpyrimidine. Both of these dihydrofolate reductase inhibitors rapidly pass the blood-brain barrier, concentrate in brain and have brain/plasma ratios of 1.3 to 2.6.[58] To the author's knowledge neither of these drugs has yet been tested in intracerebral rodent tumors.

Vincristine

Vincristine is an alkaloid isolated from the plant *Vinca rosea*. It is primarily an antimitotic agent (M-phase-specific) and behaves as such against AKR lymphoma.[8] Its mechanism of action is conceived as a reversible disruption of the tubular protein in the mitotic spindle.[59] Similarly, disruption of microtubules in peripheral nerves with the production of distal, Wallerian degeneration is thought to be the mechanism of the neurotoxicity which is the chief, dose-limiting side-effect of this agent.[60] The drug has been administered I.V. at various dose schedules ranging from 1 mg/m^2 every eight days to 1 to 1.5 mg/m^2 every two weeks.

Vincristine very rarely causes hematoxicity at the recommended doses, and for this reason, plus the fact that it is phase-specific, it is an attractive agent for use in combination chemotherapy. However, its inclusion in prospective studies will be difficult because of severe, dose-related neurotoxicity, some manifestations of which are seen in virtually every patient receiving this agent.

The neurotoxicity of this drug has been reviewed by Sandler, et al.[61] In the author's own experience, reflex abnormalities are invariably present within six weeks (two to four treatments at a dose of 1 to 2 mg/m^2) of initiating treatment. Unless the dose is reduced, loss or severe reduction of deep tendon reflexes is followed by paresthesias, gait disturbance, cranial nerve palsies, and cerebral dysfunction. Motor weakness occurred in 36 percent of Sandler's series, usually manifest as foot or wrist extensor weakness.[61] In the author's experience this is an indication for immediate cessation of therapy, as recovery is slow and often incomplete. Virtually all patients complain of disturbing paresthesias, usually in the fingertips, less often in the toes. Although in most cases no sensory loss was detected, paresthesias became the dose-limiting factor in a number of patients. Extraocular palsies are common,[61, 62] but unlike the poor recovery rate for peripheral motor weakness, recovery is usually complete within a range of three weeks to four months. Seizures and psychoses have been observed only at very high dose levels.

Cramping abdominal pain, distention, and severe constipation occur and seem more prevalent in children. Impotence is another less common but very disturbing side-effect. Alopecia of varying degrees occurs in one-half to one-third of patients.

In practice, the dose of vincristine is not lowered after loss of reflexes but will usually be cut in half if paresthesias occur and discontinued if motor weakness is noted. Although his experience is small, rarely has the author been able to reinstitute therapy after cessation. Toxic side-effects seem to become manifest earlier in patients with hepatic dysfunction. Sandler's data[61] would suggest that 2 mg/m² every week can usually be tolerated, but the author's data would indicate that schedules of administration every two weeks or on days one and eight every month are better tolerated.

Vincristine and the closely related drug vinblastine have been tested against human tumors *in vitro*.[63, 64] Shapiro failed to show an increase in survival when vincristine, administered I.P., was used in the murine intracerebral ependymoblastoma system.[65]

Many clinical studies in which vincristine was used alone or in combination have been reported. The number of patients in report is small, but if all studies are taken together, one can conclude that the effectiveness of this agent has been demonstrated. Braham[66] described four patients with recurrent, primary brain tumors who were treated with doses of .05 to .1 mg/kg every week for three months with courses repeated after a one month rest period. Improvement was noted in all cases within four to six weeks, lasting for no less than three months. Two of these patients had recurrent glioblastomas. The ability of patients to tolerate repeated courses at the dosage used without significant toxicity is unusual. In only one patient did the tendon reflexes disappear.

Lassman, et al.[61] reported twelve cases of primary brain tumors treated with weekly I.V. doses of 0.5 mg/kg. The criteria for patient selection make this a Phase III study, but the details of histologic type with respective longevity are not sufficiently clear to warrant firm conclusions. There was one clear-cut response unrelated to surgery or radiotherapy in a patient with a recurrent medulloblastoma. The authors concluded that the treatment was apparently effective in three of five cases with astrocytic glioma. This same group reported rapid improvement in bony pain due to metastatic medulloblastoma in two patients within forty-eight hours of the initial injection of .05 mg/kg.[68]

Smart, et al. presented a series of one hundred seventy-six patients with tumors of many organ systems.[69] Their data for toxicity, its severity, and time of onset, agree with the author's. They report a 25 percent response rate for all their C.N.S. tumors, but data on the relation of the start of chemotherapy to the original surgical treatment is lacking and precludes a comparison of their results with those in other series. They reported four dramatic responses including a medulloblastoma, a cervical astrocytoma, and a supratentorial tumor diagnosed as a malignant astrocytoma on the basis of an angiogram.

Mealey, et. al.[70] administered vincristine by intracarotid infusion in combination with I.A. mithramycin in seven cases, and administered the same drugs I.V. in one additional case, with no visible responses. Their patients all fitted into the context of a Phase II study and were well matched. The malignant astrocytomas from these eight patients were grown in tissue culture and then exposed to media containing vincristine and mithramycin in an unsuccessful attempt to establish a correlation between cytotoxicity *in vitro* and clinical results.

Owens, who has had the most extensive experience with I.A. vincristine against brain tumors[71, 72] summarized his work.[73] As of 1967, Phase II and Phase III patients with glioblastomas were treated by the technique of intermittent infusion of 1 to 2 mg a day to a total of from 10 to 15 mg. At that dose nausea, ileus, conjuntival erythema, and forehead erythema became dose-limiting side-effects. Of special interest is the observation that peripheral neuropathy did not occur with doses exceeding the total I.V. dose that regularly produces symptoms. Of thirty patients who received vincristine as an adjunct to surgical therapy (Phase III), four were still alive, surviving an average of thirty-five months, and the remaining twenty-six had an average postsymptom survival time of fourteen months. All patients had the histological diagnosis of glioblastoma. No separate statistics were presented for the patients with recurrent tumors. The use of survival time measured from the onset of first symptoms is unfortunate. Survival from the time of surgery would have had greater significance. Despite these encouraging results, Owens concluded that a critical review of his data leaves an impression that factors other than chemotherapy could have accounted for the results obtained.

In summary, vincristine, administered either I.V. or I.A., has produced isolated responses in the treatment of brain tumors. To date there has been no well-controlled Phase II or Phase III study. The cumulative neurotoxicity observed after I.V. administration would suggest that a Phase III study would be doomed to failure from the start if prolonged intermittent therapy is planned. Intermittent I.A. therapy also has dose-limiting side-effects plus the morbidity of chronic catheter replacement. The lack of hematoxicity and the prospect of more widely spaced therapy make this drug theoretically interesting for combination therapy, yet in the two studies so far reported,[12,70] the results have been disappointing. It is the author's feeling that more basic research with this drug, alone and in combination, in animal brain tumor models is needed before further clinical studies are warranted.

Nitrogen Mustard

Nitrogen mustard (mechlorethamine) was one of the first chemotherapeutic agents brought into clinical use[74] and the first to be tried in brain tumor patients. In subsequent studies the drug was administered by intracarotid infusion or perfusion. Woodhall and Mahaley,[75] who pioneered the technique of cerebral perfusion, summarized the results of sixty-three perfusions and one hundred ten infusions. They used a variety of drugs including nitrogen mustard, cytoxan, phenylalanine mustard, Thiotepa and several amino acid analogs. They reached the conclusion that none of these agents provided a significant prolongation of life. Of the group, nitrogen mustard proved the most toxic to the C.N.S., causing many instances of acute cerebral edema and extraocular muscle palsies. This toxicity had been observed before and studied in both animals and man by J.D. French and associates,[76] who demonstrated vascular congestion, perivascular demyelination, chronic neuronal degeneration, and cortical gliosis. Ownes[73] employed intracarotid nitrogen mustard and simultaneously gave I.V. sodium thiosulfate to neutralize the drug reaching the systemic circulation. His technique avoided both local and systemic complications, but the average posttreatment survival time in fifteen cases of glioblastoma was nine months, and he concluded that the procedure had achieved no significant prolongation of life.

Although the results were discouraging, these men did the pioneer work in brain tumor chemotherapy and provided a stimulus for further investigation of drugs and routes of administration.

Thiotepa

Thiotepa (triethylene thiophosphoramide), a compound closely related to the mustards, was another of the early agents tested. The results reported by Mahaley and Woodhall have already been mentioned.[75] Aronson et al., using[32] P-labeled Thiotepa, found no significant uptake of this compound by an intracerebral tumor.[77] It is difficult to understand why a drug of high lipid solubility could not be found in tumor, and this observation bears repetition before being accepted as fact.

Neither Thiotepa nor nitrogen mustard is being investigated at the present time.

Epodyl

Epodyl (resorcinol diglycidyl ether) is a lipid-soluble synthetic compound investigated as an anticancer agent by Imperial Clinical Industries in Great Britian in the early 1960's. It acts as an alkylating agent and has a serum half-life of ten to fifteen minutes, as do many agents in this class. After a single I.V. dose in rats, the highest tissue concentrations are found in brain, and it diffuses freely into the cerebrospinal fluid.[78] Epodyl has been shown to be cytotoxic against human astrocytomas and glioblastomas grown in culture.[79] Early clinical studies suggested a more marked therapeutic advantage when the drug was administered by I.A. rather than I.V., and the clinical brain tumor studies reported here all utilized the former technique.

In 1964 Taylor, et al.[80] reported treating thirty patients bearing large inoperable brain tumors using a dose of 75 to 100 mg/kg. Thirteen were reported alive from six months to two years after a single treatment, but many of these had grade I or II astrocytomas. Nevertheless, eight of thirty were described as showing clinical improvment unrelated to steroid administration. Unilateral facial edema, alopecia, and symptoms of acute swelling of the tumor were common side-effects.

Goracz[81] treated forty glioblastoma patients with a combination of intracarotid epodyl and radiotherapy. He reported five patients alive over two years using a schedule of 5 gm every week repeated three to four times. He commented on four unoperated patients who showed definite improvement on this regimen. These results would not seem significantly better than what would be expected from radiation alone. Steroids were also given to these patients, rendering interpretation of the results even more difficult.

The largest series reported in detail described the treatment of eighty-two patients (seventy-nine with gliomas) using a schedule of 100 to 200 mg/kg by intracarotid infusion repeated three times at monthly intervals.[82] With radiation and steroids taken into consideration, forty-six responses were reported; in five patients improvement did not occur until after the second treatment. There were five deaths attributable to drug therapy from causes other than marrow depression (e.g., carotid thrombosis, acute cerebral edema) and three patients became blind in one eye from severe chemosis. The major systemic side-effect was delayed myelosuppression with the nadir of the white blood cell count (W.B.C.) occurring at two weeks and recovery after three to five weeks. This report did not mention cumulative toxicity.

In summary, I.A. administration of epodyl has led to improvement in patients with brain tumors although the side-effects have been both frequent and serious. Its use I.V. either alone or in combination with another agent in a Phase II study would seem indicated, but at the present time the FDA I.N.D. (Federal Drug Administration Investigational New Drug) application has been withdrawn.[83]

Imidazole Carboxamides

Dimethyl triazeno imidazole carboxamide (DTIC, NSC-45388) was synthesized in 1962 and in early screening studies was shown to be effective against murine neoplasms.[84] Phase I trials demonstrated that the I.V. route of administration was most effective, and a number of Phase I and Phase II studies have been summarized.[85]

Favorable responses were observed in some cases of intracerebral metastases from malignant melanoma,[86] but totally discouraging results have been reported by others.[87] The author has used this drug in a nine day I.V. course to treat a small number of patients harboring a variety of intracerebral tumors unresponsive to prior treatment with BCNU and observed one response in eight patients.[88] Although DTIC has not received a fair clinical trial, further studies are not warranted because this agent does not penetrate the normal blood-brain barrier.[89] Further, it has no particular advantage in combination chemotherapy because, like other cycle-nonspecific agents, its dose-limiting toxicity is reflected in delayed bone marrow depression.

BIC (TIC-mustard; NSC 82196), given in doses of 900 mg/m² daily for five days every six weeks, was evaluated because of its greater lipid solubility and the fact that it showed modest activity against intracerebral glioma 26.[90] Of eighteen patients evaluated in a Phase II study, 39 percent responded; however, the median duration of response was only four months compared to nine months for BCNU.[88]

5-fluorouracil

This agent, a pyrimidine antagonist found to be effective against tumors of the colon, has been administered I.V. and applied locally to human brain tumors. The drug crosses the blood-brain barrier and is found in normal brain. A significantly large tumor-to-brain ratio of both 5-FU and its active metabolite was found in murine ependymoblastoma.[91] Bourke, et al. have recently provided data on the kinetics of entry of 5-FU into the brain and CSF of normal primates following I.V. or I.T. administration.[92]

Edland, et al.[93] randomized patients with glioblastoma to 5-FU alone and 5-FU plus radical supervoltage radiotherapy in a Phase III study. In the combined treatment regimen the 5-FU was administered I.V. thirty to sixty minutes before radiation treatment three times per week for about three weeks at a dose of 5 mg/kg. No difference in survival between the two groups was noted. Ringkjob[94] applied 5-FU soaked gelatin sponge to the tumor bed, and in some patients a catheter was left *in situ* for local infusion each day for four days after surgery. The longest survival in thirty-two patients with grade III or IV astrocytomas was six months. The *in vivo* data cited suggest that 5-FU deserves consideration for further studies to find optimal schedules and routes of delivery.

Bromouridine (BUDR)

Bromouridine (BUDR), although not itself cytotoxic, sensitizes cells to ionizing radiation. Bromouridine, a halogenated analog of thymidine, is taken up by cells as an exogenous source of thymidine. The preadministration of 5-FU or methotrexate increases cellular incorporation of BUDR, presumably by blocking intracellular thymidine synthesis and rendering the cell more dependent upon an exogenous source of thymidine.

Sano, et al.[95] developed a complicated protocol for the use of this drug in patients with malignant gliomas. BUDR and methotrexate were infused daily into the carotid artery for two weeks before and also for three to four weeks during the period of radiation therapy. Fully a quarter of the twenty-five patients treated by this technique were alive longer than one and one-half years following surgery. Despite the prolonged period that the catheter was in place, there were only four infections and only two were serious enough to require removal of the catheter. Thrombosis and embolism were not observed. This method of treatment, although complex, resulted in a significantly increased survival time for many of the patients involved.

Sano, et al. have recently reported their updated experience with this technique.[96] Having treated a total of forty-six patients bearing highly malignant gliomas they reported one year survival rates of 60 percent, two years, 36 percent, and three years, 15 percent. These results are the best yet reported for any mode of treatment for malignant gliomas. To the author's knowledge this technique has not been used in North America, but their results should stimulate research into the combined use of radiation and radiosensitizing agents.

AGENTS UNDERGOING TRIALS

Bleomycin (NSC 123506)

Bleomycin is a water-soluble antibiotic isolated in Japan from a strain of *Streptomyces verticillus*. Biochemically, it can be separated into a number of fractions of which the one designated A2 has the greatest oncolytic activity. In the commercially available preparation, the A2 fraction makes up 53 percent of total bleomycin. Animal studies suggest that bleomycin prevents cells from entering mitosis but does not prevent DNA replication.[97] Studies in Japan[98] have shown that bleomycin injected subcutaneously achieves high concentrations within a 20-methylcholanthrene-induced mouse brain tumor, but that levels in the surrounding normal brain are quite low. A great advantage of this agent is its lack of hematoxicity, making it a logical choice for combination chemotherapy.

Clinical trials in Japan, using an I.V. dosage of 15 mg every four days to a total dose of 300 mg, showed a clinical response in six of twelve patients with malignant gliomas.[98] Unfortunately, many of these patients received concurrent radiotherapy making interpretation of the response rate difficult. Takeuchi[99] treated fourteen patients with malignant gliomas using the same dose and schedule and observed responses in nine. Again in this series, the relationship of chemotherapy to surgery is unclear, and some of these patients received radiotherapy.

The side-effects of bleomycin have been reviewed.[9,100] Fever is the most common, occurring in 32 percent of cases. Anorexia, alopecia, and joint thickening in the hands were also common. The most serious side-effect, interstitial penumonitis, led to deaths in 1 percent of the Japanese combined series.[100] Fatal pulmonary complications occurred only in older patients who received total doses exceeding 300 mg.

The recommended dose is 15 mg/m² I.V. every four days for six weeks. The results reported from Japan, although inconclusive, warrant further trials in this country either as a single agent or as part of a combination protocol for primary brain tumors. One Phase II screening study already reported included two patients with glioblastoma, neither of whom showed any response.[101]

Procarbazine (NSC 77213)

Procarbazine is a derivative of methyl hydrazine which has

already proved to be an effective agent in the treatment of Hodg-kins disease.[102] It is believed to act by depolymerizing DNA and is therefore considered a cycle-nonspecific agent. It has been shown to cross the blood-brain barrier and equilibrate in the CSF.[103] Its main side-effect, acute nausea and vomiting, limits the size of daily doses. Delayed hematoxicity is the most serious toxic mani-festation, with leucopenia and thrombocytopenia appearing two to eight weeks after the start of therapy. Cessation of therapy at this time is followed by recovery of peripheral counts in one to three weeks, and thereafter a maintenance dose may be tolerated.

The author has completed a Phase II study with this agent, giving 150 mg/m^2 orally each day for thirty days.[104] A rest period of one month was followed by a second course and similarly, further courses depending on the degree and persistence of the hematoxicity. The overall response rate was 44 percent. Three of four patients with medulloblastomas responded, one for nineteen months. This response ratio indicates a degree of effectiveness similar to that obtained with either BCNU or CCNU, and makes procarbazine another potential agent for combination chemo-therapy.

Methyl-CCNU

This drug is another nitrosourea derivative very similar in structure to CCNU, which has already been discussed. More lipid soluble than CCNU, it is effective against the murine glioma.[105] Phase I studies have been carried out, and results showed re-sponses in several patients with brain tumors.[106] A cooperative Phase III trial by the BTCSG is currently in progress.

Corticosteroids

One would be remiss to conclude a detailed account of chemo-therapeutic agents without discussing corticosteroids. This should not be surprising, since no other agent has been used as frequently and as successfully in the treatment of intracerebral tumors. Thus, in the broadest terms, corticosteroids are chemo-therapeutic agents, although their modes of action have yet to be completely defined. Few would now deny the evidence, both clinical and experimental,[107, 108] that corticosteroids have a significant effect on the edema associated with both malignant primary and metastatic brain tumors, and it seems equally evident that the rapid, often dramatic clinical improvement seen in patients treated with corticosteroids is due to the reduction of this edema.

In addition, corticosteroids may possess a direct antineoplastic effect as well. There is now considerable evidence in experimental brain tumors,[109,110,111] that DNA synthesis is in some manner inhibited.[112] Corticosteroids may simply lengthen the cell cycle and thus retard tumor growth, or they may have a direct tumoricidal action; possibly they may act by a combination of these effects.

How this proposed antineoplastic action can be determined in the clinical situation is even less clear. It is obvious that one cannot randomize patients to steroids and no steroids and detect a weak antineoplastic effect, since it would be impossible to separate antiedema effects from the presumed antineoplastic effect. If corticosteroids affect the cell cycle of dividing tumor cells, they may reduce the effectiveness of phase-specific antineoplastic agents. Corticosteroids are believed to act on the cell membrane, and it is also possible that they can favorably or unfavorably affect the entry of chemotherapeutic agents into the cell.[113] Kinetic studies, both in animals and humans, will be needed to answer these questions. Until then, corticosteroids will continue to be used primarily for their antiedema action, and thus as adjuncts to other chemotherapeutic agents.

COMBINATION CHEMOTHERAPY

The most significant advances in clinical chemotherapy during the past decade have resulted from the use of combinations of agents, together or in sequence, in the treatment of leukemias and lymphomas.[114,115] There is every reason to believe that the same approach will lead to improved results in the treatment of brain tumors.

Many theories have been put forward to explain the failure of single agent therapy, one or several of which may be applicable in any particular case. The most important of these are as follows: (1) At the time of treatment, especially in the case of recurrent tumors, the mass is large and presumably a much lower percentage of cells are in cycle than when the tumor was smaller, blood supply was adequate, and cell crowding was not a factor of importance. In such cases, treatment with phase-specific agents will not effect a significant cell kill and in fact the drug, whether phase- or cycle-specific, may not be able to penetrate to susceptible areas. (2) Many tumors, including glioblastomas, are composed of two or more tumor cell types. Different tumor cell types may have different sensitivities to oncolytic agents. In this case the tumor volume may be reduced temporarily at the expense of a susceptible type, but as resistant types continue to proliferate, the tumor mass will return to and then surpass its original size. (3) In addition, a susceptible line of tumor cells may, after repeated exposure, become gradually resistant. There is evidence that this occurs with methotrexate.[116]

Theoretically, drug combinations can counteract such problems in the following ways: (1) The use of a cycle-specific agent to reduce the bulk of a tumor followed by a phase-specific agent which will be effective against an increasing proportion of cycling cells has been applied to experimental systems.[117] Only because of advances in the understanding of tumor population kinetics has such an approach become possible (see Chapter Two). (2) By using drugs which manifest their toxic side effects in different organ systems, it is usually possible to administer each drug at full dose. (3) By using two or more agents it may be possible to reduce the frequency of exposure to any one agent so that the development of resistance will be delayed or prevented. (4) It is possible that certain drugs in combination will have an additive or synergistic effect. It is, of course, equally possible that certain drug combinations will be antagonistic.

The successful application of combination protocols to brain tumor chemotherapy has two essential prerequisites. First, it would seem obvious that drugs selected for combination therapy should be those agents proven useful in single drug trials. In this regard, additional drugs must be found which have the therapeutic efficacy of BCNU and procarbazine and/or which offer another advantage in the form of different toxicity. Second, prior to clinical application, combinations of theoretical advantage should be evaluated in animal systems to determine optimal dose-schedule relationships. The author's own clinical combination studies of BCNU-vincristine[12] and procarbazine-CCNU-vincristine[118] were not preceded by critical experiments in animal models.

In the BCNU-vincristine study, BCNU was administered 90 mg/m² daily for three days every six to eight weeks and vincristine 0.5 mg/kg one day a week. In twenty patients the addition of vincristine provided no advantage over BCNU alone.

In a subsequent study of procarbazine, CCNU, and vincristine (PCV), procarbazine was given 100 mg/m² every day for fourteen days, CCNU 100 mg/m² in a single dose, and vincristine 1.4 mg/m2 on days one and eight; the sequence was repeated at four to six week intervals depending on toxicity. The response rate in the PCV study was comparable to responses achieved with BCNU, CCNU, or procarbazine alone; moreover, the number of long-term responders seemed greater than those witnessed with other protocols, and the response of medulloblastomas was four out of four with long-term responses continuing at three months.

These studies employing combination drug therapies for malignant brain tumors represent a modest beginning. At present the combined use of BCNU and procarbazine, the two most effective agents in single drug trials, is being explored. In the future, combined modality approaches to brain tumors will be pursued with the conviction that surgery, radiotherapy, chemotherapy, and possibly immunotherapy must be combined to significantly improve the treatment of malignant gliomas.

REFERENCES

1. Greene, M.O. and Greenberg, J.: The activity of nitrosoguanidines against ascites tumors in mice. *Cancer Res, 20*:1166, 1960.
2. Schabel, F.M., Jr., Johnston, T.P., McCaleb, G.S., et al.: Experimental evaluation of potential anticancer agents. VIII. Effects of certain nitrosoureas on intracerebral L1210 leukemia. *Cancer Res, 23*:725, 1963.
3. Rall, D.P. and Zubrod, C.G.: Mechanisms of drug absorption and excretion. Passage of drugs in and out of the central nervous system. *Ann*

Rev Pharmacol, 2:109, 1962.

4. Wilkoff, L.J.: Kinetic evaluation of the effect of agents interfering with DNA synthesis on viability of cultured leukemia L1210 cells. *Proc Am Assoc Cancer Res, 12*:8, 1971.

5. Loo, T.L., Dion, R.L., Dixon, R. L., and Rall, D.P.: The antitumor agent, 1,3-bis(2-chloroethyl)-1-nitrosourea. *J Pharm Sci, 55*:492, 1966.

6. Groth, D.P., D'Angelo, J.M., Vogler, W.R., et al.: Selective metabolic effects of 1,3-bis(2-chloroethyl)-1-nitrosourea upon *de novo* purine biosynthesis. *Cancer Res, 31*:332, 1971.

7. Wheeler, G.P. and Bowdon, B.J.: Some effects of 1,3-bis(2-chloroethyl)-1-nitrosourea upon the synthesis of protein and nucleic acids *in vivo* and *in vitro*. *Cancer Res, 25*:1770, 1965.

8. Bruce, W.R. and Valeriate, F.A.: Normal and malignant stem cells and chemotherapy. In: *The Proliferation and Spread of Neoplastic Cells*. A collection of papers presented at the Twenty-First Annual Symposium on Fundamental Cancer Research, Baltimore, Williams & Wilkins, 1968, pp. 409-422.

9. Shapiro, W.R., Ausman, J.I., and Rall, D.P.: Studies on the chemotherapy of experimental brain tumors: evaluation of 1,3-bis(2-chloroethyl)-1-nitrosourea, cyclophosphamide, mithramycin, and methotrexate. *Cancer Res, 30*:2401, 1970.

10. DeVita, V.T., Denham, C., Davidson, J., and Oliverio, V.T.: The physiological disposition of the carcinostatic 1,3-bis(2-chloroethyl)-1-nitrosourea (BCNU) in man and animals. *Clin Pharmacol Ther, 8*:566, 1967.

11. Rall, D.P., Ben, M., and McCarthy, D.M.: 1,3-bis-chloroethyl-1-nitrosourea (BCNU): toxicity and initial clinical trial. *Proc Amer Assoc Cancer Res, 4*:55, 1963.

12. Fewer, D., Wilson, C.B., Boldrey, E.B., et al.: The chemotherapy of brain tumors. Clinical experience with carmustine (BCNU) and vincristine. *JAMA, 222*:549, 1972.

13. Walker, M.D. and Hurwitz, B.S.: BCNU (1,3-bis(2-chloroethyl)-1-nitrosourea; (NSC-409962) in the treatment of malignant brain tumor — a preliminary report. *Cancer Chemother Rep, 54*:263, 1970.

14. Walker, M.D. and Gehan, E.A.: An evaluation of 1-3-bis(2-chloroethyl)-1-nitrosourea (BCNU) and irradiation alone and in combination for the treatment of malignant glioma. *Proc Am Assoc Cancer Res, 13*:67, 1972.

15. Hansen, H., Selawry, O.S., Muggia, F.M., and Walker, M.D.: Clinical studies with 1-(2-chloroethyl)-3-cyclohexyl-1-nitrosourea (NSC 79037). *Cancer Res, 31*:223, 1971.

16. Levin, V.A., Shapiro, W.R., Clancy, T.P., and Oliverio, V.T.: Uptake, distribution and antitumor activity of 1-(2-chloroethyl)-3-cyclohexyl-1-nitrosourea (CCNU) in the murine ependymoblastoma. *Cancer Res, 30*:2451, 1970.

17. Swenberg, J.A.: Treatment of primary brain tumors with CCNU. *Proc Am*

Assoc Cancer Res, 14:25, 1973.

18. Walker, M.D., Rosenblum, M.L., Smith, K.A., and Reynolds, A.F., Jr.: The treatment of brain tumor with 1-(2-chloroethyl)-3-cyclohexyl-1-nitrosourea (CCNU). *Proc Amer Assoc Cancer Res, 12*:51, 1971.

19. Fewer, D., Wilson, C.B., Boldrey, E.B., and Enot, K.J.: Phase II study of 1-(2-chloroethyl)-3-cyclohexyl-1-nitrosourea (CCNU;NSC-79037) in the treatment of brain tumors. *Cancer Chemother Rep*, part I, *56*:421, 1972.

20. Rosenblum, M.L., Renynolds, A.F., Jr., Smith, K.A., et al.: Chloroethyl-cyclohexyl-nitrosourea (CCNU) in the treatment of malignant brain tumors. *J Neurosurg, 39*:306, 1973.

21. Yarbro, J.W., Kennedy, B.J., and Barnum, C.P.: Mithramycin inhibition of RNA synthesis. *Cancer Res, 26*:36, 1966.

22. Northrop, G., Taylor, S.G., III, and Northrop, R.L.: Biochemical effects of mithramycin on cultured cells. *Cancer Res, 29*:1916, 1969.

23. Medrek, T.: Personal communication. April, 1968.

24. Ransohoff, J., Martin, B.F., Medrek, T.J., et al.: Preliminary clinical study of mithramycin (NSC-24559) in primary tumors of the central nervous system. *Cancer Chemother Rep, 49*:51, 1965.

25. Brown, J.H. and Kennedy, B.J.: Mithramycin in the treatment of disseminated testicular neoplasms. *N Engl J Med, 272*:111, 1965.

26. Kofman, S.: Mithramycin, an antibiotic used in cancer chemotherapy. *Proc Am Assoc Cancer Res, 5*:36, 1964.

27. Kofman, S. and Eisenstein, .R.: Mithramycin in the treatment of disseminated cancer. *Cancer Chemother Rep, 32*:77, 1963.

28. Kennedy, B.J., Brown, J.H. and Yarbro, J.W.: Mithramycin (NSC-24559) therapy for primary glioblastomas. *Cancer Chemother Rep, 48*:59, 1965.

29. Kennedy, B.J., Yarbro, J.W., Kickertz, V., and Sandberg-Wollheim, M.: Effect of mithramycin on a mouse glioma. *Cancer Res, 28*:91, 1968.

30. Wilson, C.B. and Barker, M.: Relative cytotoxicity of mithramycin and vinblastine sulfate in cell culture of human neural tumors. *J Natl Cancer Inst, 38*:459, 1967.

31. Medical News: Neurosurgeons collaborate in study of brain tumor drugs. *JAMA, 210*:240, 1969.

32. Whitside, J.A., Philips, F.S., Dargeon, H.W., and Burchenal, J.H.: Intrathecal amethopterin in neurological manifestations of leukemia. *Arch Intern Med, 101*:279, 1958.

33. Levin, V.A., Clancy, T.P., and Ausman, J.I.: Methotrexate permeability and steady-state distribution in the murine ependymoblastoma. *Trans Am Neurol Assoc, 94*:294, 1969.

34. Tator, C.H.: Chemotherapy of brain tumors. Uptake of tritiated methotrexate by a transplantable intracerebral ependymoblastoma in mice. *J Neurosurg, 37*:1, 1972.

35. Anderson, L.A., Collins, G.J., Ojima, Y., and Sullivan, R.D.: A study of the distribution of methotrexate in human tissues and tumors. *Cancer Res, 30*:1344, 1970.

36. Rubin, R., Owens, E., and Rall, D.: Transport of methotrexate by the choroid plexus. *Cancer Res, 28*:689, 1968.
37. Rall, D., Rieselbach, R., Oliverio, V., and Morse, E.: Pharmacology of folic acid antagonists as related to brain and cerebrospinal fluid. *Cancer Chemother Rep, 16*:187, 1962.
38. Condit, P.: Studies on the folic acid vitamins. II. The acute toxicity of amethopterin in man. *Cancer, 13*:222, 1960.
39. Capizzi, R.L., DeConti, R.C., Marsh, J.C., and Bertino, J.R.: Methotrexate therapy of head and neck cancer: improvement in therapeutic index by the use of leucovorin "rescue". *Cancer Res, 30*:1782, 1970.
40. LeVitt, M., Nixon, P., Pincus, J., and Bertino, J.: Transport characteristics of folates in cerebrospinal fluid. A study utilizing double-labeled 5-methyltetrahydrofolate and 5-formyltetrahydrofolate. *J Clin Invest 50*:1301, 1971.
41. Blair, J.A. and Searle, C.E.: Reversal of methotrexate toxicity in mice by 5-methyltetrahydrofolic acid. *Br J Cancer, 24*:603, 1970.
42. Goldin, A., Venditti, J.M., Kline, I., and Mantel, N.: Eradication of leukaemic cells (L1210) by methotrexate and methotrexate plus citrovorum factor. *Nature (Lond), 212*:1548, 1966.
43. Hakala, M.T., Zakrzewski, S.F., and Nichol, C.A.: Relation of folic acid reductase to amethopterin resistance in cultured mammalian cells. *J Biol Chem, 236*:952, 1961.
44. Hryniuk, W.M. and Bertino, J.R.: Treatment of leukemia with large doses of methotrexate and folinic acid: clinical-biochemical correlates. *J Clin Invest, 48*:2140, 1969.
45. Levitt, M., Mosher, M.B., DeConti, R.C., et al.: Improved therapeutic index of methotrexate with "leucovorin rescue." *Cancer Res, 33*:1729, 1973.
46. Ojima, Y. and Sullivan, R.D.: Pharmacology of methotrexate in the human central nervous system. *Surg Gynecol Obstet, 125*:1035, 1967.
47. Norrell, H., Jr.: Personal communication. September, 1971.
48. Shapiro, W.R., Chernik, N.L., and Posner, J.B.:Nicrotizing encephalopathy following intraventricular instillation of methotrexate. *Arch Neurol, 28*:96, 1973.
49. Bleyer, W.A., Drake, J.C., and Chabner, B.A.: Neurotoxicity and elevated cerebrospinal-fluid methotrexate concentration in meningeal leukemia. *New Engl J Med, 289*:770, 1973.
50. Watkins, E., Jr. and Sullivan, R.D.: Cancer chemotherapy by prolonged arterial infusion. *Surg Gynecol Obstet, 118*:3, 1964.
51. Sayers, M.P.: Intrathecal methotrexate therapy of brain tumors of childhood. *Ohio State Med J, 65*:383, 1969.
52. Rubin, R.C., Ommaya, A.K., Henderson, E.S., et al.: Cerebrospinal fluid perfusion for central nervous system neoplasms. *Neurology (Minnaep), 16*:680, 1966.
53. Weiss, S.R. and Raskind, R.: Treatment of malignant brain tumors by local methotrexate. *Int Surg, 51*:149, 1969.

54. Norrell, H. and Wilson, C.: Brain tumor chemotherapy with methotrexate given intrathecally. *JAMA, 201*:15, 1967.
55. Wilson, C.B. and Norrell, H.A.: Brain tumor chemotherapy with intrathecal methotrexate. *Cancer, 23*:1038, 1969.
56. Skeel, R., Cashmore, A., and Bertino, J.: Pre-clinical trials of a new triazine antifolate, NSC 139105. *Proc Am Assoc Cancer Res, 14*:52, 1973.
57. Levin, V.: Unpublished observations.
58. Stickney, D.R., Simmons, W.S., DeAngelis, R.L., et al.: Pharmacokinetics of pyrimethamine (PRM) and 2,4-diamino-5-(3′, 4′-dichlorophenyl)-6-methylpyrimidine (DMP) relevant to meningeal leukemia. *Proc Am Assoc Cancer Res, 14*:52, 1973.
59. Palmer C.G., Livengood, D., Warren, A.K., et al.: The action of vincaleukoblastine on mitosis *in vitro*. *Exp Cell Res, 20*:198, 1960.
60. Schlaepfer, W.: Vincristine-induced axonal alterations in rat peripheral nerve. *J Neuropath Exp Neurol, 30*:488, 1971.
61. Sandler, S.G., Tobin, W., and Henderson, E.S.: Vincristine induced neuropathy. A clinical study of fifty leukemic patients. *Neurology (Minneap), 19*:367, 1969.
62. Albert, D.M., Wong, V.G., and Henderson, E.S.: Ocular complications of vincristine therapy. *Arch Ophthalmol, 78*:709, 1967.
63. Chen, T.T. and Mealey, J., Jr.: The responses of malignant gliomas to combination chemotherapy *in vitro*. *Proc Amer Assoc Cancer Res, 12*:71, 1971.
64. Chen, T. and Mealey, J., Jr.: Microculture of human brain tumors. *Cancer Chemother Rep, 54*:9, 1970.
65. Shapiro, W.R.: Studies on the chemotherapy of experimental brain tumors. Evaluation of 1-(2-chloroethyl)-3-cyclohexyl-1-nitrosourea, vincristine, and 5-fluorouracil. *Natl Cancer Inst Monogr, 46*:359, 1971.
66. Braham, J., Sarova-Pinhas, I., and Goldhammer, Y.: Glioma of the brain treated by intravenous vincristine sulphate. *Neurochirurgia (Suttg), 12*:195, 1969.
67. Lassman, L.P., Pearce, G.W., and Gang, J.: Sensitivity of intracranial gliomas to vinblastine sulphate. *Lancet, 1*:296, 1965.
68. Lassman, L.P., Pearce, G.W., Path, M.C., et al.: Vincristine sulphate in the treatment of skeletal metastases from cerebellar medulloblastoma. *J Neurosurg, 30*:42, 1969.
69. Smart, C.R., Ottoman, R.E., Rochlin, D.B., et al.: Clinical experience with vincristine (NSC-67574) in tumors of the central nervous system and other malignant diseases. *Cancer Chemother Rep, 52*:733, 1968.
70. Mealey, J., Chen, T.T., and Pedlow, E.: Brain tumor chemotherapy with mithramycin and vincristine. *Cancer, 26*:360, 1970.
71. Owens, G.: Chemotherapy of brain tumors. In: Krayenbuhl, H., Maspes, P.E., and Sweet, W.H. (Eds.): *Progress in Neurol Surgery*. Basel, Karger, 1966, vol. I, pp. 190-201.
72. Owens, G., Javid, R., Tallon, M., et al.: Arterial infusion chemotherapy of

primary gliomas. *JAMA, 186*:802, 1963.

73. Owens, G.: Intraarterial chemotherapy of primary brain tumors. *Ann NY Acad Sci, 159*:603, 1969.

74. Rhoads, C.P.: Nitrogen mustards in the treatment of neoplastic disease. *JAMA, 131*:656, 1946.

75. Malaley, M.S., Jr. and Woodhall, B.: Regional chemotherapeutic perfusion and infusion of brain and face tumors. *Ann Surg, 166*:266, 1967.

76. French, J.D., West, P.M., von Amerongen, F.K., and Magoun, H.W.: Effects of intracarotid administration of nitrogen mustard on normal brain and brain tumors. *J Neurosurg, 9*:378, 1952.

77. Aronson, H.A., Flanigan, S., and Mark, J.B.D.: Chemotherapy of malignant brain tumors using regional perfusion. I. Technic and patient selection. *Ann Surg, 157*:394, 1963.

78. *Epodyl Review.* Imperial chemical industries. Mereside Alderley Park, 1969.

79 Easty, D.M. and Wylie, J.A.: Screening of 12 gliomata against chemotherapeutic agents *in vitro. Br Med J, 1*:1589, 1963.

80. Bailey, I.C., Taylor, A.R., and Grebbell, F.S.: Ethoglucid in treatment of inoperable cerebral tumors. *Br Med J, 1*:1161, 1964.

81. Goracz, I.: The combined treatment of glioblastoma multiforme. *Minerva Neurochir, 13*:248, 1969.

82. Khanna, H.L., Bailey, I.C., Taylor, A.R., and Grebbell, F.S.: Epodyl in the management of cerebral glioma. *Neurology (Minneap), 19*:570, 1969.

83. Jewell, J.B.: Personal communication. December, 1970.

84. Shealy, Y.F., Montgomery, J.A., and Laster, W.R.: Antitumor activity of triazenoimidazoles. *Biochem Pharmacol, 11*:674, 1962.

85. Luce, J.K., Thurman, W.G., Isaacs, B.L., and Talley, R.W.: Clinical trials with the antitumor agent 5-(3,3-dimethyl-1-triazeno) imidazole-4-carboxamide (NSC-45388). *Cancer Chemother Rep, 54*:119, 1970.

86. Burke, P.J., McCarthy, W.H., and Milton, G.W.: Imidazole carboxamide therapy in advanced malignant melanoma. *Cancer, 27*:744, 1971.

87. Skibba, J.L., Ramirez, G., Beal, D.D., and Bryan, G.T.: Preliminary clinical trial and the physiologic disposition of 4(5)-(3,3-dimethyl-1-triazeno) imidazole-5(4)-carboxamide in man. *Cancer Res, 29*:1944, 1969.

88. Wilson, C.B., Gutin, P., Kumar, A.R.V., et al.: Single chemotherapy of brain tumors: a five-year review. (in preparation).

89. Vogel, C.: Pharmacologic and immunologic studies with a new anti-tumor agent, imidazole-4(or 5)-carboxamide, 5 (or 4) 3,3-bis(2-chloroethyl)-1-triazeno (NSC 82196). *Proc Amer Assoc Cancer Res, 10*:96, 1969.

90. Levin, V.A., Hansch, C., Wilson, C.B., et al.: Imidazole carboxamides: structure-activity relationships in intracerebral glioma 26 and human brain tumors. *Cancer Chemother Rep 59*:327-331, 1975.

91. Levin, V.A. and Chadwick, M.: Distribution of 5-fluorouracil-2-^{14}C and its metabolites in a murine glioma. *J Natl Cancer Inst, 49*:1577, 1972.

92. Bourke, R.S., West, C.R., Chheda, G., and Tower, D.B.: Kinetics of entry

and distribution of 5-fluorouracil in cerebrospinal fluid and brain following intravenous injection in a primate. *Cancer Res, 33*:1735, 1973.

93. Edland, R.W., Javid, M., and Ansfield, F.J.: Glioblastoma multiforme — an analysis of the results of postoperative radiotherapy alone versus radiotherapy and concomitant 5-fluorouracil. *Am J Roentgenol Radium Ther Nucl Med, 111*:337, 1971.

94. Ringkjob, R.: Treatment of intracranial gliomas and metastatic carcinomas by local application of cytostatic agents. *Acta Neurol Scand, 44*:318, 1968.

95. Sano, K., Hoshino, T., and Nagai, M.: Radiosensitization of brain tumor cells with a thymidine analogue (Bromouridine). *J Neurosurg, 28*:530, 1968.

96. Sano, K., Hatanaka, H., Takakura, K., and Nagai, M.: *Combined Chemo-radio-therapies in the Treatment of Malignant Brain Tumors.* Presented to the American Association of Neurological Surgeons, Boston, Mass. April 17, 1972.

97. Nagatsu, M., Okagaki, T., Richart, R.M., and Lambert, A.: Effects of bleomycin on nuclear DNA in transplantable VX-2 carcinoma of rabbit. *Cancer Res, 31*:992, 1971.

98. Kanno, T., Nakazawa, T., and Kudo, T.: ²Study of Bleomycin on Brain Tumors. Publication of the School of Medicine, Keio University, Tokyo, Japan, 1970.

99. Takeuchi, K.: *Effects of Bleomycin on Brain Tumors.* Presented at the thirty-first meeting of the Kanto District of Japan Neurological Society, November 29, 1969.

100. Statistical Observation of the Side Effects of Bleomycin. Publication of the Fuse National Hospital, Tokyo. ref. II, 48, 1968.

101. Shastri, S., Slayton, R., Wolter, J., et al.: Clinical study with bleomycin. *Cancer, 28*:1142, 1971.

102. Stodinsky, D.C., Solomon, J., Pugh, R.P., et al.: Clinical experience with procarbazine in Hodgkin's disease, reticulum cell sarcoma, and lymphosarcoma. *Cancer, 26*:984, 1970.

103. Oliverio, V.T.: Pharmacologic disposition of procarbazine. In Carter, S.K. (Ed.): *Proceedings of the Second National Cancer Institute (NCI) New Drug Seminar; Chemotherapy Conference on Procarbazine (Matulane NSC-77213): development and application, Bethesda, Md., 1970.* Bethesda, U.S. Govt. Printing Office, 1971, pp. 19-28.

104. Kumar, A.R.V., Renaudin, J., Wilson, C.B., et al.: Procarbazine hydrochloride in the treatment of brain tumors. Phase II study. *J Neurosurg, 40*:365, 1974.

105. Carter, S.: From a paper presented at the Second Joint Working Conference, NCI Chemotherapy Program, Annapolis, Maryland, November 3-5, 1971.

106. Young, R.C., Walker, M.D., Canellos, G.P., et al.: Initial clinical trials with methyl-CCNU 1-(2-chloroethyl)-3-(4-methyl cyclohexyl)-1-

nitrosourea (MeCCNU). *Cancer, 31*:1164, 1973.

107. Lippert, R.G., Svien, H.J., Grindlay, J.H., et al.: The effect of cortisone on experimental cerebral edema. *J Neurosurg, 17*:583, 1960.

108. Long, D.M., Hartmann, J.F., and French, L.A.: The response of human cerebral edema to glucosteroid administration. An electron microscopic study. *Neurology (Minneap), 16*:521, 1966.

109. Wright, R.L., Shaumba, B., and Keller, J.: The effect of glucocorticosteroids on growth and metabolism of experimental glial tumors. *J Neurosurg, 30*:140, 1969.

110. Gurcay, O., Wilson, C.B., Barker, M., and Eliason, J.: Corticosteroid effect on transplantable rat glioma. *Arch Neurol, 24*:266, 1971.

111. Kotsilimbas, D.G., Meyer, L., Berson, M., et al.: Corticosteroid effect on intracerebral melanomata and associated cerebral edema. Some unexpected findings. *Neurology (Minneap), 17*:223, 1967.

112. Chen, T.T. and Mealey, J., Jr.: Effect of cortisteroid on protein and nucleic acid synthesis in human glial tumor cells. *Cancer Res, 33*:1721, 1973.

113. Zager, R.F., Frisby, S.A., and Oliverio, V.T.: Cellular transport and antitumor activity of methotrexate (MTX) in combination with clinically useful drugs. *Proc Amer Assoc Cancer Res, 13*:33, 1972.

114. Burchenal, J.H.: Success and failure in present chemotherapy and the implication of asparaginase. *Cancer Res, 29*:2262, 1969.

115. Carter, S.: Clinical trials and combination chemotherapy. *Cancer Chemother Rep*, part 3, *2*:81, 1971.

116. Borsa, J. and Whitmore, G.F.: Cell killing studies on the mode of action of methotrexate on L-cells *in vitro*. *Cancer Res, 29*:737, 1969.

117. Strauss, M.J., Mantel, N., and Goldin, A.: The effect of the sequence of administration of cytoxan and methotrexate on the life-span of L1210 leukemic mice. *Cancer Res, 32*:200, 1972.

118. Gutin, P., Wilson, C.B., Kumar, A.R.V., et al.: Phase II study of procarbazine, CCNU, and vincristine combination chemotherapy in the treatment of malignant brain tumors. *Cancer 35*:1398-1404, 1975.

CHAPTER **EIGHT**

CONCLUSION

CHARLES B. WILSON

AS THIS MONOGRAPH goes to press, it is tempting to postpone publication in order to incorporate exciting laboratory and clinical investigations currently in progress. The same thought must plague other authors writing on subjects in similar states of rapid evolution. This author will refer briefly to ongoing research in projecting the future direction of brain tumor chemotherapy.

The preceding chapters present the principles upon which current and future research must build to achieve the ultimate objective of curing human gliomas. Here have been presented kinetic parameters determined from a series of malignant gliomas, and I am convinced that this information is imperative for selecting drugs and for designing administration schedules, particularly for multiagent therapy. Pharmacokinetic data is equally important in selecting potentially useful agents and their most appropriate route and schedule. In all probability, continued experiments in animal models will produce more efficient screens for new drugs, and the role of such models in research on multiple therapeutic modalities is already evident.

Experience with clinical trials served as the basis for Chapters Five and Six. Patient selection and subsequent evaluation of their response to chemotherapy constitute the foundations of Phase II trials, and in the foreseeable future the identification of active agents, singly and in combination, will depend upon properly designed and executed Phase II trials. As the chemotherapy coordinator has assumed increasing responsibility for patient care, her role has become essential in this author's program. Miss Enot defines this role in Chapter Six. Because patients harboring brain tumors have problems unique to their disease, her experience in coordinating their care both in and out of the hospital will serve as a valuable guide to nurses and paramedical personnel involved with brain tumor chemotherapy.

In the immediate future several areas of promising research can be seen. Animal models will be used to explore surgery, irradiation, and chemotherapy in various combinations and sequences. On the bases of data related to cell population kinetics, pharmacokinetics, the time course of DNA injury and repair, and the log reduction of clonogenic cells achieved by each modality, the author hopes to design curative multiple modality therapy. We anticipate that improved animal screens will identify more effective agents for Phase II clinical trials.

The search for biologic markers will continue. Logically, such a marker should be present in cerebrospinal fluid. Its value would lie not so much in initial diagnosis as in its use as an accurate biochemical means by which to follow the course of patients during treatment.

Many investigators are pursuing clinical immunotherapy, and trials with human patients harboring primary brain tumors are evolving. Ultimately immunotherapy will become one component of multiple modality therapy.

Never has the future of brain tumor chemotherapy been more optimistic. More than anything else, the field needs bright young investigators. The authors of this monograph will be abundantly repaid if they have recruited even a few neophytes to a field in which the task is enormous and the workers too few.

APPENDIX A

Examples of Instruction and Information Sheets
given to patients receiving BCNU in the Chemotherapy Service
University of California Medical School

BCNU has a delayed effect. Its activity begins at about two or three weeks after treatment, and its effect is noticed by the patient at about four or five weeks after administration.

Blood counts *must* be done as instructed below. It is imperative that the reports be sent immediately to:

Charles B. Wilson, M.D.
Department of Neurological Surgery
University of California Medical Center
San Francisco, Ca. 94143

The blood counts are to be done every Monday and Thursday. The necessary counts are complete blood count (c.b.c.) and platelet count.

The reason for the blood counts is that BCNU does have the side-effect of depressing blood counts in a fairly predictable pattern. At about three weeks after treatment, the platelet counts will drop, and then will usually spontaneously rise after one or two weeks. Then, just as the platelet count rises, the white blood cell count will fall, and will stay low for about two weeks. The effects noticeable to the patient during these drops are:

Low platelet count — very easy bruising, possible bleeding from the nose and, very rarely, blood may be noted in the urine. If any bleeding occurs, call your local physician immediately, and also contact Jean Enot.
Low white blood cell count results in increased susceptibility to infection.

You will be notified by Jean Enot or your physician if your counts have reached a level dangerous to you.

159

The time interval between courses of BCNU varies with the course of treatment. Return admission appointments will be scheduled before your hospital discharge. For help with any questions, or should you need immediate help, do not hesitate to call Jean Enot. Phone numbers: 666-1087 (office)
Jean Enot: 863-1947 (home)

Dr. Wilson can also be reached through the office number evenings and on weekends.

Be patient, have your blood counts done, and we will see you soon.

Instructions and information for
patients receiving Procarbazine®

Procarbazine is given orally. On the initiation of treatment with Procarbazine and BCNU, Procarbazine will be given on days 2 through 15 and days 30 through 43. Thereafter, it will be given for 21 consecutive daily doses and with similar 21 day courses beginning the day after each dose of BCNU. The dates to be given will be written in below.

Lab studies to be done during the course of treatment are:

C.B.C. and platelet count — every Monday and Thursday.

SGOT, alkaline phosphatase, and urinalysis — every Monday.

These reports are to be sent immediately to:

Charles B. Wilson, M.D.
Department of Neurological Surgery
University of California Medical Center
San Francisco, California 94143

Symptoms of toxicity from this drug are multiple. They include: nausea and vomiting, diarrhea, constipation, headache, extreme fatigue, cough, nosebleed, and changes in the blood.

Dietary restrictions are: no alcohol, cheese, or bananas.

Medicine restrictions are: no sleeping pills, antihistamines, or tranquilizers.

Should the family or patient at any time become alarmed by any of the side-effects or by the patient's condition, DO NOT HESITATE to notify the coordinator or Dr. Wilson.

APPENDIX B

UNIVERSITY OF CALIFORNIA

Consent to Act as Subject for
Research and Investigations

Subject's Name:_____, Date: _____

(1) I hereby authorize _____
(Name of person(s) who will perform the procedure(s)

and/or investigation(s) and/or any such assistants as may be selected by him) to perform the following procedure(s) and/or in-
vestigation(s):

The Procarbazine capsule(s) are given at bedtime for a period of
30 days. The first dose or two of each course will be given in the
hospital, in order that antinausea drugs can be given for the
nausea and vomiting which often accompanies the first several
doses. After 30 days of treatment there is a rest period of 30 days
after which the patient returns to the hospital to begin his second
course. Blood counts and blood chemistries will be drawn twice
weekly, and urinalysis is performed once a week during the 30
days of treatment; all tests are done during the 30 day rest period
also.

The dietary restrictions are: no cheese, bananas, or alcohol.
Medication restrictions are: no tranquilizers, sleeping pills, or
antihistamines.

(2) The procedure(s) and/or investigation(s) listed in paragraph (1) has (have) been explained to me by _____

(Name)

(3) I understand that the procedure(s) and/or investigation(s)
described in paragraph (1) involves (involve) the following possible risks and discomforts ....

Nausea and vomiting often accompany the first several doses of
each course. These complications are alleviated and sometimes

prevented by antinausea medications, but in some cases therapy must be stopped because of intractable nausea or vomiting.

A drop in the white blood count and/or platelet count occurs frequently. These changes in the blood cells can lead to serious and potentially fatal infections or bleeding disorders. Less common but annoying side-effects include diarrhea, constipation, loss of appetite, muscle and joint pains, cough, itching, chills, fatigue, and mouth sores.

(4) I understand that the combined use of the above medications is experimental, and may or may not be of benefit to me.

(5) I understand that _____
              (Name of person(s) who will perform procedure(s) and/or

_____
investigation(s) and/or such assistants as may be selected by him) will answer any inquiries I may have at any time concerning the procedure(s) and/or investigation(s).

(6) I understand that I may terminate my participation in the study at any time, and that, owing to the scientific nature of the study, the investigator may in his absolute discretion terminate my participation at any time.

(7) I understand that my termination of participation in this study will in no way jeopardize my relationship with _____ or the neurological surgery service or the brain (the physician) tumor chemotherapy service.

                           _____
                           Subject's Signature

                           _____
                           Witness

UNIVERSITY OF CALIFORNIA

Consent to Act as Subject for
Research and Investigation

Since no person may legally consent to research procedures to be done on any other person, this signature is not legally binding. It does indicate, however, that you are aware of this research and agree to it. Without your signature, the investigator will not do the study on the person in question.

Subject is a minor age_____
Subject is unable to sign for self because _____
_____

Father _____
Mother _____
Guardian _____

APPENDIX C

Subject's Name: _____
Date:_____

(1) I hereby authorize _____
(Name of person(s) who will perform
_____
the procedure(s) and/or investigation(s) and/or any such assistants as may be selected by him (to perform the following procedure(s) and/or investigation(s):

Because no known conventional form of treatment following partial surgical excision of my tumor has proved more effective than another, my treatment selection will be made by NIH investigators who will at the time of treatment selection consider the number of patients assigned to each treatment selection and arbitrarily decide my treatment.

I will receive one of the following treatment regimens:

1. Methyl-CCNU, an oral antitumor drug
2. Methyl-CCNU and radiation therapy
3. BCNU, an intravenous antitumor drug, and radiation therapy
4. Radiation therapy

Methyl-CCNU is given by mouth once every 6 to 8 weeks. If it is given in combination with radiation therapy, the first course of methyl-CCNU is given 1 to 7 days before the start of radiation therapy, and the second course is given after the completion of radiation therapy when the blood counts have returned to near normal or normal levels. Subsequent courses of methyl-CCNU are given at 6 to 8 week intervals, depending on the recovery of the

165

blood counts.

The procedure for radiation therapy will be explained to me by Dr. Glenn Sheline and/or his associates.

BCNU, an antitumor drug, is given by intravenous drip once a day for three days over a 30 to 45 minute period within 1 to 7 days before starting radiation therapy. The second course of BCNU is given after the completion of radiation therapy, and when the blood counts have returned to normal or nearly normal levels. The BCNU treatment is repeated thereafter at 6 to 8 week intervals, depending on the return of blood counts to normal or nearly normal levels.

I understand that the treatment selection may or may not be of benefit to me.

(2) The procedure(s) and/or investigation(s) listed in paragraph (1) has (have) been explained to me by:

_____

(3) I understand that the procedure(s) and/or investigation(s) described in Paragraph (1) involves (involve) the following possible risks and discomforts:

Methyl-CCNU

Nausea and vomiting are common 3 to 12 hours following treatment. Antiemetics are helpful but not necessarily preventive in alleviating this discomfort.

A drop in the white blood cell count and/or platelet count occurs consistently. These changes in the blood cells can lead to serious and potential fatal infections or bleeding disorders.

Damage to the kidneys, liver, heart, and lungs has been observed in experimental animals, but this has not been a problem in humans.

In order to monitor closely the effects on the blood, I will have blood studies done according to the methyl-CCNU information sheet.

The risks of radiation therapy will be explained to me by Dr. Glenn Sheline and/or his associates. It is possible that the combination of methyl-CCNU or BCNU and radiation therapy may have more effect on my blood than either treatment alone.

BCNU

The infusion of BCNU may give local pain and/or a burning sensation in the arm of injection during the time of infusion only. Often 20 to 40 minutes after receiving BCNU, I may notice a temporary (20 to 45 minutes) flushing of my face. About 50 percent of the patients may have nausea and/or vomiting 3 to 12 hours after completion of the infusion; this stops in less than 24 hours. Antinausea medication will be given to lessen or stop the vomiting.

A drop in the white blood cell count and/or platelet count occurs consistently. These changes in the blood cells can lead to serious and potentially, although highly unlikely, fatal infections or bleeding observed in experimental animals, but this has not been observed in humans. In order to monitor closely the effects of BCNU on the blood, I will have blood studies done according to the BCNU information sheets.

I understand that the benefits are as follows:

Treatment is designed to kill and/or slow the regrowth of tumor left behind after operation, although in my case treatment may be of no value.

(4) I understand that _____

(Name of person(s) who will perform

_____

procedure(s) and/or investigation(s) and/or such assistants as may be selected by him) will answer any inquiries I may have at any time concerning the procedure(s) and/or investigation(s).

(5) I understand that I may terminate my participation in the study at any time, and that, owing to the scientific nature of the study, the investigator may in his absolute descretion terminate my participation at any time, and that this will in no way jeopardize my relationship with the Neurosurgery Service or the Chemotherapy Service.

(6) I am not aware that_____

Patient's Name

has ever expressed a desire that he would not wish experimental therapy.

UNIVERSITY OF CALIFORNIA

Consent to Act as Subject for
Research and Investigations

Since no person may legally consent to research procedures to be done on any other person, this signature is not legally binding. It does indicate, however, that you are aware of this research and agree to it. Without your signature, the investigator will not do the study on the person in question.

Subject is a minor age ⎯⎯⎯⎯⎯⎯⎯

Subject is unable to sign for self because ⎯⎯⎯⎯⎯⎯⎯⎯⎯⎯

⎯⎯⎯⎯⎯⎯⎯⎯⎯⎯⎯⎯⎯⎯⎯⎯⎯⎯⎯⎯⎯⎯⎯⎯⎯⎯⎯⎯⎯⎯

Father ⎯⎯⎯⎯⎯⎯⎯⎯⎯⎯⎯

Mother ⎯⎯⎯⎯⎯⎯⎯⎯⎯⎯⎯

Guardian ⎯⎯⎯⎯⎯⎯⎯⎯⎯

APPENDIX D

Instructions for Patients Receiving Methyl-CCNU Chemotherapy

Methyl-CCNU is a delayed-action chemotherapeutic agent; it begins at about four weeks after treatment. Improvement will probably not be noted until four to six weeks after treatment.

The side-effect of methyl-CCNU is bone marrow depression; for this reason twice weekly blood counts must be done. The counts necessary are: c.b.c. and platelet counts. These tests are to be done every Monday and Thursday. It is imperative that the reports are sent upon completion to:

> Charles B. Wilson, M.D.
> Department of Neurological Surgery
> University of California Medical Center
> Third and Parnassus
> San Francisco, Ca. 94143

Noticeable effects of the bone marrow depression are bruising, pallor, and fatigue. These are transient and normal responses.

Extreme reaction to methyl-CCNU may be seen by bleeding from the bladder, nose, or bowels. This reaction must be reported immediately to your local physician and to Jean Enot or Dr. Wilson. Extremely severe drops in blood counts, or severe bleeding may be treated with blood transfusions.

Additional laboratory studies that must be done, and the schedule for these are as follows:

First and second weeks after treatment: SMA-12 Panel once weekly

Third and fourth weeks after treatment: SMA-12 Panel and urinalysis twice weekly

Fifth, and succeeding weeks: SMA-12 Panel once weekly

169

If any problems arise, or the patient's condition changes suddenly, please contact Jean Enot or Dr. Wilson as soon as possible.
Telephone Numbers: Dr. Wilson: 666-1087
Jean Enot: 666-1087
home number: 863-1947

APPENDIX E

HUMAN SUBJECTS SECTION

(1) Requirements for Subject Population

Our studies pertain to brain and C.N.S. tumor patients only. Children are often treated if they meet the study requirements, but they are not necessarily treated as a special group. Frequently, brain tumor patients are not mentally competent due to their disease. Every effort is made to assure that they fully understand treatment procedures so that they can give informed consent. At times, next of kin must make the decision as to whether or not to proceed with treatment.

(2) Potential Risks

All chemotherapy side-effects are outlined in the protocol and are discussed with the patient in advance. The greatest risk involves depressed blood counts, which are closely monitored during treatment. All side-effects and risks are presented in writing and are thoroughly discussed with the patient and responsible next of kin. Other methods of treatment (e.g. surgery, radiotherapy) also involve risks, and the patient has the option of choosing the form of treatment, or no treatment. Diseases being treated are uniformly fatal without treatment.

(3) Consent Procedures

Consent to treat with chemotherapy is discussed with the patient and responsible next of kin by the chemotherapy nurse. Consent in writing is obtained after the patient has been evaluated as eligible for chemotherapy, has been informed of alternatives to chemotherapy, and after he has verbally expressed a desire for this form of treatment. The patient understands that he may withdraw from the study at any time or may be removed from the study by the investigator, if necessary.

(4) Protecting Against Risks

The patient and his family have open communication lines at all times with the chemotherapy nurse and the physicians. Blood counts are monitored closely, and results are sent to our department twice a week. The patient is also followed between treatments by his private physician, if he lives too far away for our physicians to examine him. In the event of severe or unusual side-effects, treatment can be stopped or altered. Letters and hospitalization reports are sent to the referring physicians and those involved in posttreatment care.

(5) Potential Benefits

It is quite possible that the patients will have decreasing tumor sizes along with increasing mental and physical functions as a result of chemotherapy. The possibility of elimination of the tumor also exists. The long-range goal to benefit society is to control growth of and, hopefully, cure brain tumors.

(6) Risk-Benefit Ratio

Since the diseases we treat are uniformly fatal without therapy, any form of effective therapy, even if it is palliative, is welcome. The risks of life-threatening leukopenia or thrombocytopenia are small and usually controllable.

APPENDIX F

June 23, 1972
TO: Deans, Directors, Department Chairmen, Principal Investigators
FROM: Committee on Human Experimentation

Attached are three items which the campus Committee on Human Experimentation hopes will expedite and facilitate the review process of projects involving humans as research subjects. These three items are:

(a) A cover sheet providing for certain detailed information which should be attached to and a part of every submission of a protocol to the Academic Senate office, 506 U.

(b) A fairly long document entitled, "Advisory Letter to Investigators." This document presents in a condensed form most of the material present in the new HEW guidelines published under date of December 1, 1971*. In addition, it contains advice on the preparation of protocols which the local Committee believes will expedite review and will reduce the amount of correspondence back and forth between the Committee and the investigators.

(c) Attachment (A) is the regular consent form to serve as a research subject as prepared in the General Counsel's office. As indicated in the Advisory Letter to Investigators, this consent form should be used in all experimental projects unless a specific modification of it or an exemption is authorized by the Committee on Human Experimentation. The attached form has had deleted the section for signature

---

*(The HEW guidelines referred to are entitled, "The Institutional Guide to DHEW Policy on Protection of Human Subjects". This is DHEW publication #(NIH) 72-102, and it is available from the Superintendent of Documents, United States Government Printing Office, Washington, D.C. 20402 for 25¢ per copy (Stock #1740-2302).

by parents. This form can be signed only by an individual 18 years old or older who is legally competant to sign for himself or herself. If the use of minors is contemplated, consult with the Senate office or the Committee chairman regarding the additional section required on the form.

The consent form makes provision for specifying patient compensation in case of failure to complete a study. The local Committee requires the full amount of compensation to be specified in addition.

ADVISORY LETTER TO INVESTIGATORS
FROM: COMMITTEE ON HUMAN EXPERIMENTATION

The Department of Health, Education and Welfare (DHEW) has issued guidelines for human experimentation, which were published on December 1, 1971. In these guidelines each institution is charged with the responsibility for safeguarding the rights and welfare of the human subjects involved in experiments. The institution must set up a committee on human experimentation (CHE) to review all studies involving human experiments to determine that:

(1) the rights and welfare of the subjects are adequately protected;

(2) the risks to the individual are outweighted by the potential benefits to that individual or the importance of the knowledge gained; and

(3) informed consent is obtained by methods that are appropriate and adequate. In addition, the CHE must establish a basis for continuing review of activities involving human experimentation.

The DHEW guidelines state:

"An individual is considered to be 'at risk' if he may be exposed to the possibility of harm — physical, psychological, sociological, or other — as a consequence of any activity that goes beyond the application of those established and accepted methods necessary to meet his needs. The determination of when an individual is at risk is a matter of the application of common sense and sound professional judgment to the circumstances of the activity in question. Responsibility for this determination resides at all levels of institutional and departmental review. Definitive determination will be made by the operating agency."

From this it is clear that the risk inherent in routine diagnostic and therapeutic measures done only for the patient's benefit is not the concern of the CHE. What the CHE is concerned about is the health, welfare, and safety of individuals who may be at risk as a consequence of participation as a patient or subject in research, development, demonstration, or other activities supported by the University.

There are several types of risk. The most obvious is physical harm; for example, nerve injury during attempted venipuncture; arterial thrombosis after an arterial catheterization; a drug reaction. Then there can be psychological harm with mental or physical consequences; for example, depression or other mental disturbance after an interview that arouses strong emotions. Social harm can occur if the results of the test or interview cause embarassment or public humiliation. Finally there may be legal risks; for example, the finding of metabolites of heroin in urine, the finding of XXY karyotype in blood taken for some other purpose. Therefore risk can occur when something is done to a subject, to material taken from a subject in the course of normal medical care or even from examination of medical records. Retrospective examination of medical records, especially those many years old, probably does not cause harm provided confidentiality is preserved.

Definition of an Experiment

What constitutes an experimental procedure? Clearly an established and accepted diagnostic or therapeutic procedure done for the benefit of the patient is not an experiment. This procedure requires the informed consent of the patient, e.g. signed consent for general anesthesia, but is no concern of the CHE. Any activity where a patient or subject may be at risk as a result of his or her participation which does not conform to the above description is an experiment which must receive prior CHE approval, and these fall into three groups:

Class 1 — A diagnostic or therapeutic procedure done for the benefit of the patient upon whom it is practiced but departing from accepted or established standards of medical management for that patient. Note that a procedure may be accepted and standard in Europe but not in California; its use in California would therefore be regarded as experimental.

Class 2 — An experiment done on an unhealthy individual with the intention of discovering more about some aspect of the illness. Here the intent is to obtain knowledge, not to diagnose or treat the patient's illness. The patient could possibly benefit from the results of the study but usually no immediate benefit is expected.

Class 3 — An experiment done on normal people.

Confusion exists when the experiments are done as part of routine care. If subjects are allocated to groups at random, that is clearly an experiment. If data are analyzed to provide answers to questions, that is an experiment. If a procedure is done elsewhere as part of routine care but, because of unsolved questions, further study is done here, that constitutes an experiment. Consider patients being given one or both of two drugs and having blood levels measured at various intervals. If the decision about which drugs to give and what samples to measure is purely part of medical management, but the data are going to be analyzed to determine if one drug affects the blood levels of the other, then all that is needed is that confidentiality be preserved. If blood is removed in addition to that needed for routine management or if in the blood samples measurements are made of substances not usually measured for management of the patient, then this must be explained and consent given for use of the added samples or measurement of the additional substances. If one of the drugs would not be given normally, then permission for its use must be obtained.

If the experimenter has any doubts about whether the procedure is an experiment, the protocol must be submitted to the CHE. The members of the CHE or the experts they consult may find risks that were not considered by the investigator. Not only is this important because it is required by DHEW, but it also helps protect the patient against harm as well as protecting the investigator, the University, or other sponsor against legal action should harm occur.

Scope of CHE Activities

Prior approval by the CHE is required for any human experiments done:

(i) with funds administered by the University of California, no matter what the source of those funds, or

(ii) in any of the institutions used by or affiliated with the University of California, or

(iii) at the University of California or in any of the institutions used by or affiliated with the University of California *even when no funds are involved.*

Prior approval by the CHE is not needed for human experiments done without funds supplied by or administered by the University of California and conducted off the University and its affiliated premises when the investigator acts in his capacities as a private citizen, in his capacity as a staff member of another hospital or research organization, and is not acting as a staff member, employee, or agent of the University of California. However, the investigator must apprise the CHE of any such experiment and certify that he is not acting as a staff member, employee, or agent of the University while conducting such an experiment.

Aids to Efficient Protocols

With these points in mind, the investigator can help himself and the CHE by drawing up an efficient protocol. This must include the following, although some aspects may not apply to certain protocols:

(1) Emphasize the importance of the project for the patient or for others. This will help the CHE to assess the balance of risks and benefits.

(2) If applicable, state what has already been done in animals and describe why further animal study is not appropriate.

(3) How will subjects be selected? This helps the CHE to decide if there are any special risks for that group. In addition, there must be added concern for the protection of

those in prison, in mental institutions, those subject to military discipline, and those in schools or colleges. It is important to be sure that no subjects, whether patients or not, are coerced or improperly induced in any way to join the study.

(4) The number of subjects studied, the duration of the study and an indication of the method of analysis are required. While the CHE does not set itself up in judgment of the scientific merit of the study, any study that seems manifestly incapable of answering the questions posed could be considered as one in which the risks exceed the benefits. You should state whether the subjects will be used in more than one experiment.

(5) Any reimbursement to subjects should not be excessive and should be justified. This prevents enticing subjects to go against their better judgment. Nominal reimbursement for time and discomfort is reasonable.

(6) The risks must be stated as completely as possible, especially if the procedure used is more than a simple venipuncture or if any drugs are given. The risks will have to be considered relative to the group studied. Thus, might the drug affect pregnant women? the elderly? those with renal impairment? those driving cars? If certain rare complications have been observed, but only in higher doses than those contemplated, this must be mentioned. The more detail provided, the easier it will be to assess the application. Incomplete statements are among the commonest reasons for return of the application to the investigator with consequent waste of time for all concerned.

(7) Will the study be done in the hospital or on ambulatory subjects? Will the risks be reduced by doing the study in the hospital?

(8) Will the subjects be under the care of a physician other than the investigator? It is important that a physician be available to advise the subject about any contraindications to the study and be available to request that the study be stopped prematurely if it is not in the subject's interest to continue. In general, the investigator should arrange for a

physician not involved in the study to perform this function. In practice, this may not always be possible; the investigator must then specify in detail what would lead to cessation of the study. If there is an uninvolved physician, the investigator should state who it will be. Clearly there is little protection for the subject if this physician is a junior Fellow who might not be willing to offend the senior investigator.

(9) If new drugs are to be used, there must have been an application to the FDA for use of an I.N.D. (Investigational New Drug). Under the provisions of the Federal Food, Drug, and Cosmetic Act, as amended in 1962, and the California Pure Drug Act of 1965, a "new" drug is a substance or preparation not generally recognized by qualified experts as being safe and effective for the use proposed. A drug may be "new" without necessarily being a new substance. Even an accepted remedy, used for years, is considered to be a "new" drug if it is not generally recognized as being safe and effective for the proposed new use or the new dosage. Thus the Food and Drug Administration, though recognizing a given drug or drug product (i.e., the active material in its final dosage form) as safe and effective for certain well-defined medical uses, may consider it to be a new drug if the drug product is altered in any of the following ways:

   (i)   The intended use or dose is different from the officially recognized or approved.
   (ii) The route of administration is different from that officially approved.
   (iii) The dosage form (including components and their quantities) is different from that officially approved.
   (iv) New scientific evidence relative to the safety and/or efficacy of the drug or drug product comes to light.

Often when a new or investigational drug is being used in a study, the pharmaceutical company will file an I.N.D. application. However, the proposed study must conform with the protocol submitted and approved by the FDA.

Any change from the submitted protocol requires review by the FDA and by the CHE.

Approval by the FDA of the experimental use of a new drug does not excuse the CHE from deciding on its safety, and the CHE may request the investigator to supply relevant information about the safety and function of the new drug.

Occasionally the investigator may wish to use a drug preparation not cleared by the FDA as a research tool, for early clinical investigations of a drug for a new therapeutic or diagnostic use, or in a new dosage form of a previously used drug. The investigator must submit sufficient evidence to the CHE to satisfy them of the safety of the drug under the proposed circumstances. The CHE may require the investigator to complete the Food and Drug Form #1571 and to submit the data to the FDA for their approval.

(10) The use of radio-isotopes in experiments must be approved by the Radio-isotope Safety Committee. The CHE should be given a copy of their approval.

(11) If major diagnostic procedures are used (e.g. arteriography, biopsy) the investigator must make clear if these are done for the study or if the patient would of necessity have had them for his routine medical care.

(12) How consent is to be obtained and the manner in which consent is to be determined must be included in all protocols.

Informed Consent

Many applications are rejected because of inadequate consent forms, or because the consent of the subject will not be obtained by a method that is adequate. All medical treatment, except an emergency in which the patient's life is in jeopardy, requires the consent of the patient. Obviously one cannot consent to that which he does not understand, thus the term "informed consent." Before undertaking the proposed procedure, the physician owes a duty to the patient to:

(a) inform him fairly of the diagnosis and prognosis;

(b) describe in lay terms the proposed therapy;

(c) disclose fairly the risks and complications; and

(d) inform him of the results that may be anticipated.

When the proposed procedure is other than "established," generally accepted as routine medical management of the patient, the procedure becomes experimental. The requirements for the patient's informed consent remain the same, with the added precaution that the patient must be told why the physician is deviating from established practice, and the added requirement that CHE approval of the procedure, including the consent, must be obtained.

Parents, spouses, next of kin, and guardians have no legal authority to consent to experiments on patients who are not competent to consent for themselves, although they may consent to established, accepted diagnostic or therapeutic procedures done for the patient's benefit if the consent of the patient cannot be obtained. Any experimental procedure done on an individual who is unconscious, incapable of understanding the procedure, or under 18 years of age will not be legally sanctioned. It is possible that the experimenter and the University or other sponsor may be the subject of a legal suit for battery. There is ample precedent for this.

Because of the serious legal and ethical problems raised when the subjects are not legally competent to consent to experiments on themselves, some guidelines will be offered.

In Class 1 experiments where the procedure is done for the patient's benefit, permission must be obtained from the parent, spouse, next of kin, or legal guardian. This is principally for the protection of the physician who must, however, realize that the patient or relative could sue for damages should some real or fancied harm occur and is entitled to sue even if no harm is suffered. This differs from the risks incurred in routine medical management in that the absence of any negligence would not be a defense, but the absence of negligence would mitigate any claim for damage, both actual or fanciful, and thus the investigator must be prepared to defend his use of the experimental procedure.

Neither Class 2 nor Class 3 experiments should be done on individuals who cannot give informed consent. The CHE will in certain instances, however, permit research on such individuals.

Class 2 experiments pose the greater problems. The CHE recognizes that if we are to gain knowledge that will help the mentally ill, the unconscious and sick children, some research will have to be done on these subjects. For example, no matter how much work is done with human growth hormone on adults or on animals, there comes a time when experiments will have to be done on children with growth hormone deficiency if we are to advance. The proper management of fluid and electrolyte disturbances in babies would not be as advanced as it is if the distribution of water and electrolytes in normal babies had not been established. The CHE does not wish to prevent research into these fields, but the investigator who wishes to do such research must be aware of the legal hazards, and that these hazards may persuade the CHE not to approve the proposal. There is at present no legal sanction for experiments on children; they are not parental property and parents cannot legally consent to experiments on their children. Clearly new legislation is urgently needed to ensure that research into childhood illness is not severely impeded by these legal problems. Until it is enacted, however, investigators should be most careful with any approved Class 2 or 3 experiments on children lest they find themselves and the University or other sponsor involved in an indefensible legal suit for damages. In addition, investigators must recognize that it is the CHE's responsibility to determine whether the University should sponsor the particular research proposal in light of the risk to the particular patient or subject and the risk to the University. Neither the CHE nor the Office of the General Counsel desires to immobilize scientific and medical research. But in order to preclude court decisions from arising which might render certain types of research impossible, the CHE must necessarily be prudent in granting permission for research on subjects who legally cannot consent to the procedure.

    (a) Many consent forms proposed have contained the words "I therefore request ..." or "of my own free will ..." or the equivalent. These words cannot appear, since the request is usually by the investigator.

    (b) Often there has been proposed an exculpatory clause such as "I hereby release Dr. X from the consequences ..." This is expressly forbidden by DHEW, and in any event the waiving of rights probably has no force in law.

(c) The consent form must not include the possibility of the procedure helping the patient unless this is indeed true and likely. Otherwise it holds out false hope and is an illegal inducement.

(d) Consent of the patient to treatment, routine or experimental, need not be in writing to be legally effective. Indeed most medical procedures are undertaken upon oral consent. The problem with oral consent is evidentiary — attempting to establish months or even years later what was in fact said by both parties. Thus it is that a written consent which merely states, "Dr. Jones has explained the risks to me and I consent to them" is valueless if the actual statement by the physician is not documented in the experimenter's, the University's, or other sponsor's records. Accordingly, the greater the potential hazard to the patient and the greater the deviation from established or routine procedures, the more detailed the explanation to the subject, his parents or guardians should be. Therefore, the CHE will require a written statement with each protocol of the entire explanation that is proposed if the experimenter does not intend to rely on a written consent form which contains a full description of all the elements of informed consent.

(e) There are times when signed informed consent is not obtainable. Some studies are done in cultures very different from our own. In some of these cultures signed statements are regarded with suspicion, and insistence on them might make the study impossible. Examples of this might be a primitive community in Asia or Africa, or a study done on heroin addicts in this country. In these circumstances, in addition to the other requirements, the investigator must submit a statement of how he or she will explain the study to the people to obtain oral consent and this statement must be included in the protocol admitted to the CHE. When this is done, a witness to the discussion should be present.

(f) Investigators who use themselves as experimental subjects are not exempted from obtaining CHE approval and in particular must sign an informed consent form which has been reviewed and approved by the CHE. In the rare event of serious harm resulting from the experiment, the heirs might sue the University; the nature of the consent form would be important in any legal action.

(g) Generally, except for Class 1 cases, consent forms for experiments should be separate from the standard hospital forms that are used to give consent for diagnostic and therapeutic procedures, operative procedures, anesthesia, etc. In the case of Class 1 procedures, a standard hospital form may be used if the investigator has received CHE approval of the oral statement he intends to give to the patient, parent, or guardian. In Class 3 cases, no hospital forms are to be used. Use of hospital forms in Class 2 cases will depend on the factual circumstances. Some institutions, including the University, have standard forms for experimental studies. These are acceptable only if they comply with all the requirements set out in this document. The university standard forms have the approval of the General Counsel although they may not be acceptable for each and every proposal.

So much for the undesirable elements of the consent form. What is required is:

(1) A fair explanation of the procedures to be followed, including an identification of those that are experimental. These procedures must be explained in terms that the subject can understand. Any technical terms should have their lay equivalents, if necessary.

(2) There must be a description of the attendant discomforts and risks. It is appropriate to include risks and mention that these have been rare and only seen in larger doses than those to be used; these risks cannot be omitted because the investigator does not think them likely.

(3) In Class 1 cases there must be a disclosure of the appropriate alternative procedures that would be advantageous for the subject.

(4) Any benefits to be expected for the subject must be included

if they indeed exist.

(5) There must be an offer to answer the subject's questions and there should be a place where these can be set out with the replies.

(6) There must be a statement that the subject can withdraw from the study at any time without prejudice to his usual medical care, class standing, etc. Also that the subject can consult any other physician at any time concerning the study and the desirability of continuing or stopping it.

(7) When remuneration is offered to a subject, the amount of the remuneration must be specified in the consent form. In addition, provision must be made for partial remuneration in the event the subject elects to exercise his option to withdraw from the study prior to his completion (see attached consent form as prepared by the General Counsel's Office).

(8) Attachment A is the regular University of California form for consent to act as subject for research investigation as prepared in the Office of the General Counsel. In accordance with the directive from the President's Office, the Committee will require that this form be used unless the investigators justify on an individual project basis any deviation from it. This form also serves as a model in indicating all the desired elements necessary for securing informed consent.

The description of the risks needs further comment. Almost certainly any procedure that is normally harmless might on very rare occasions cause serious complications. Thus a venipuncture could conceivably introduce infection of an unusual organism to which the subject was uniquely defenseless and which could cause death. Or a skin test could by some as yet unreported mechanism cause serious late complications. Since we can never predict all these possibilities, a fully informed consent would strictly have to include some blanket sentence stating that on rare occasions the study might cause the subject's death. This is clearly unreasonable. What must be put down is the likelihood of any specific complications known to have resulted from that procedure or drug. It is appropriate to write, "Although there are no known ill effects of this (procedure) (drug), they are possible." It is appropriate to write (if true), "I understand that this procedure is frequently done for (diagnostic) (therapeutic) purposes and that the complications described to me are rare." It would be appropriate to have a general statement to the effect that the usual precautions will be taken.

The investigator is advised to consider having an uninvolved physician present when the consent form is discussed with the subject. This physician can attest that the risks were fairly discussed with the subject and can be available for discussion of the procedures with the subject.

AUTHOR INDEX

SUBJECT INDEX

A

Administration, routes of, *see* Drug administration
Agents, *see* Drugs
AKR lymphoma, 12
 chemotherapy of, 12-13
 see also Animal models
Amethopterin, 132
 administration of, I. T., 132
Animal models, xiii, 3-4, 10, 82-92, 157
 agents tested in, 82-83
 AKR lymphoma, 12-13
 cell kinetics of, 90-92
  calculation of, 91
  categories of, 91
  drug schedules and, design of, 90, 92
  parameters of, rat glioma, 91-92
  see also Cell kinetics
 cell loss factor in, 31
 criteria for, 84, 87
 development of, 3-4
  prewar, 3
 drug assays in, 4, 6, 88-90, 92
  BCNU, 88-89, Table 4-I, 89
  CCNU, 90
  corticosteroids, 89-90
  irradiation and, 90
  L-asparaginase, 90
  vincristine sulfate, 90
 drug effectiveness and, prediction of, 10-11
 experiments in, xiii
 glial tumor models, intracerebral, 83-85
  agents tested against, 84
  basis of, 83
  mouse glioma models for, use of, 85
  production technique for, 83-84, 85
  rat brain tumor model, new, 85-87
  rat model drug assays in, 88-90
 irradiation effects on, 90

L 1210 leukemia, 4, 82
rat brain tumor model, new, 85-87
 advantages of, 87
 characteristics of, 86
 culture of, continuous, 87
 development of, 85
 drug assays in, 88-90
 histology of, change in, 86-87
 procedure for transplantation of, 85-86
 symptoms of, 86
 tumor takes of, percentage of, 86
research in, basic, 11-12, 12-13
 AKR lymphoma, 12-13
 L 1210 leukemia, 12
Tumor growth characteristics of, 6
tumor systems used for, 10, 82-83
use of, 14, 82, 92, 158
Antifolates, 131, 136
 Amethopterin, 132
 Methotrexate, 131-136
 NSC 139105, 136
 see also Methotrexate
Arabinosyl cytosine, 13
 dose response vs toxicity results of, 13
Astrocytoma, 33
 anaplastic, 34
  labeling index for, 34-35
 astrocytes in, pilocytic, 35
 cell loss in, 37
 characteristics of, 37
 excision of, surgical, 37
 generation time of, calculation of, 33
 growth fraction of, 37
 labeling index of, 33, 34
  observed and true, 37
 S period of, 37
 studies of, histological, 37
 turnover time in, 35, 37
8-Azaguanine, 75
 assay of, *in vitro*, 75-76